Watch Your Back

Nine Proven
Strategies to
Reduce Your Neck
and Back Pain
Without Surgery

Ken Hansraj, MD

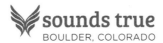
sounds true
BOULDER, COLORADO

Sounds True
Boulder, CO 80306

Sounds True is a trademark of Sounds True, Inc.

Published 2022

Book design by Charli Barnes
Illustrations © 2022 Gary Crumpler

Printed in Canada

BK06471

Library of Congress Cataloging-in-Publication Data
Names: Hansraj, Ken, author.
Title: Watch your back : nine proven strategies to reduce your neck and
    back pain without surgery / Ken Hansraj, M.D.
Description: Boulder, CO : Sounds True, 2022. | Includes index.
Identifiers: LCCN 2022011049 (print) | LCCN 2022011050 (ebook) | ISBN
    9781683649564 (hardcover) | ISBN 9781683649571 (ebook)
Subjects: LCSH: Backache--Exercise therapy. | Backache--Physical therapy. |
    Neck pain--Exercise therapy. | Neck pain--Physical therapy.
Classification: LCC RD771.B217 H358 2022
(print) | LCC RD771.B217 (ebook)
    | DDC 617.5/6406--dc23/eng/20220329
LC record available at https://lccn.loc.gov/2022011049
LC ebook record available at https://lccn.loc.gov/2022011050

10 9 8 7 6 5 4 3 2 1

This book is dedicated to my wife Marcia and
son Jonathan for their endless support.

Medical Disclaimer

This book presents the research, experiences, and ideas of its author. It is not intended to be a substitute for consultation with a professional healthcare provider. Consult with your healthcare provider before starting any program.

The author and publisher specifically disclaim all responsibility for any liability, loss, or risk, personal or otherwise, which is incurred as a consequence, directly or indirectly, of the use and application of any of the contents of this book.

The examples, anecdotes, and characters appearing in case vignettes in this book are drawn from the author's clinical work, research, and life experiences. Some are composites, and all names and some identifying characteristics have been changed throughout the book.

Contents

A Surgeon's Mission

Many people will tell you that if you consult a surgeon for medical advice, surgery is the inevitable outcome. Nothing could be further from the truth in my practice. I have been an orthopedic spine surgeon for more than twenty years. I have seen between 35,000 and 40,000 patients with complaints of back and neck pain. In the span of those two decades, I have performed 4,000 surgical procedures for some of my patients to correct their back problems. That's right—only 10 percent of the people I have treated have had to undergo surgery.

After years of studying and treating the spine, I am still awed by the brilliance of the spine's engineering and architecture. It truly is a tower of power. I have dedicated my life to keeping spines healthy and fully functional. I cannot express how rewarding it is to help my patients solve their back problems and to see how their lives change when the pain goes away.

Witnessing the suffering of my patients motivated me to develop the Watch Your Back program, which has helped to reduce back and neck pain and prevent reoccurrence for thousands of my patients. The comprehensive Watch Your Back program involves nine strategies for promoting spine health. These strategies address the physical, mental, and emotional factors that contribute to back problems. The Watch Your Back program will give you the tools you need to strengthen your back and to make your spine supple. My added focus on the psychological and emotional causes and effects of back pain has helped my patients build the confidence and strength to rise above their back problems.

I have seen how back pain prevents my patients from fully engaging in their lives. Their movement is limited, and restful sleep can be hard to get. The disruptions produced by acute or chronic pain raise their level of stress, which only exacerbates their suffering. Almost without exception, people afflicted with back pain are eager—often desperate—to find relief that does not involve prescription painkillers or surgery. My program is designed to do just that.

If you are like most people, you take better care of your car than your spine, which is at the core of your well-being. I know that our culture does not make it easy to take care of your back. You might sit at your desk all day at work, feel the stress of your demanding schedule, eat the highly processed foods that are available everywhere, or have trouble getting a good night's sleep. As you will learn, all of these can lead to back pain. The pace of life today can distract you from watching your back. My hope is to provide you with good choices and the tools to help you boost the health of your spine without disrupting your day-to-day life.

Most people are not aware of spinal health until it is gone. You should be aware of several early warning signs of an unhealthy spine, including:

- Stiffness in your back and neck

- Poor posture

- Not being able to take a satisfying, deep breath without discomfort

- A constant feeling of tension in your muscles or joints

- Your neck or back cracks when you move

- Being unable to twist or turn your head or hips to either side easily or equally

- Experiencing headaches, backaches, tender or sore spots in your joints or muscles

- Your heels wear out unevenly

- Your foot flares out when you walk

- One leg appears shorter than the other

- Poor sleep

- Feeling fatigued and just not right

An unhealthy spine gives subtle warning signs before chronic symptoms appear. Any one of these signs can be symptomatic of spinal imbalance, which may affect your overall health, vitality, and quality of life. If your spine is out of alignment, it can trigger hormonal imbalances, mood changes, lower energy, and an intensified response to stress. If you experience any of the warning signs I have listed, it is time to take action. Your spine is demanding attention. The Watch Your Back program will help you to restore your spine to optimal health.

The Watch Your Back program is meant to protect and stabilize your spine. From spinal strengthening to nutrition, from posture fixes to the power of positivity, the program consists of nine strategies you can use for pain relief and healing. Though I have published many papers in scientific journals and have written and contributed chapters to textbooks, I want to make my Watch Your Back program available to the 31 million Americans who experience back problems at any given time.

The program has worked for thousands of my patients, and I believe it will do the same for you. This book covers everything you need to know to improve the health of your spine and to reduce back pain without medication or surgery. When the program begins to work for you and your spinal health improves, you will want to make my Watch Your Back program a permanent part of your life.

Ken Hansraj, M.D.

Introduction

If Your Back Goes Out More than You Do: My Plan for Pain Relief and Healing

I f you are reading this book, I assume that you or someone you love suffers from back problems. You are far from alone. Back pain is one of the most common health complaints in the country, second only to the common cold. I use the term *back pain* in a general sense. When I refer to back pain, I mean the entire length of the spine, which includes the neck. Four out of five Americans will develop back problems in their lifetimes. I am sorry to say that more than half that number experience chronic pain for five years or more. The affliction is global. Affecting an estimated 577 million people, back problems are the leading cause of disability worldwide, while 290 million people are suffering with neck pain.

I know there is little consolation in numbers. Though many are in the same boat as you and others might "feel your pain," only you are experiencing that pain. You alone must cope with your condition and try to keep the pain from holding you back, from limiting you. You may have forgotten what it feels like to move freely with a flexible and supple spine. A healthy back supports pain-free movement. When your spine is properly aligned, you have the flexibility and mobility needed for functional movement, such as getting out of bed, going up and down stairs, and bending to pick something up. I have written this book to help you manage your pain, quell flare-ups, and avoid episodes in the future.

Watch Your Back examines what contributes to back and neck pain and what is in your power to correct. Because my program goes beyond the physical, I deal with issues you might never have connected to the back problems you experience. You might have noticed that your back acts up when you are under a lot of stress, but do you know why? Do you know how to reduce the effects of stress on your back? Do you know how to minimize acute back pain without medication? Do you know what foods and vitamins will calm inflamed nerves and muscles? Do you know what a good night's sleep will do to improve your condition? Do you know how to adjust your mindset toward your bad back to free yourself from self-imposed restrictions, which are often unnecessary? You will find the answers to these questions and more in these pages. My goal is to provide you with remedies to save you from surgery, to relieve your pain, and to protect you from relapses once the pain has resolved. In addition, the program is a necessity for rehabilitating the back after spine surgery.

The book is divided into two parts. The first covers everything you need to know about back and neck pain, from triggers to back problems to the anatomy of what can go wrong. I explain the causes of back pain and the forces you might not be aware of that put extra pressure on your spine, including posture, fashion choices, obesity, being sedentary, and bad movement. The section ends with a brief introduction to the anatomy of the spine and the physical roots of back pain.

Part 2 gives you the tools you need to watch your back, and I dedicate a chapter to each of the nine strategies for relief from back pain. I explain the significance of each strategy and give you clear instructions on how to make it a part of the way you live. Posture corrections, breathing, good movement, spinal strengthening and flexibility, nutrition for a healthy back, and getting restorative sleep are the physical components of the program. Positivity and calmness through meditation comprise the psychological and emotional aspects.

I put it all together in two daily programs created for early birds and night owls. One size does not fit all when it comes to energy highs and lows. If you routinely stay up late and have trouble getting out of bed in the morning, the chances of your doing a quick workout when you wake up are slim. If you are full of energy on waking, lag toward the end of the day, and fall into bed early, exercising before dinner would be a challenge. The daily schedules of the two programs consider when you are likely to have the most energy. Following the right Watch Your Back program for your biorhythm will make it easier for you to incorporate the program into your daily life.

Of course, you can do parts of the program whenever they work for you, your schedule, or your mood. If you have a stressful morning, you might want to meditate during your lunch break to get yourself back on track. If your partner criticizes something you have done, you might need a bit of positive thinking right away. That said, I have found that it is easier to make these practices habitual by following a regular schedule, so that the planning is already done. But life being what it is, the unexpected happens and flexibility is important. The goal is to turn to these strategies when you need them and when it is convenient. That way you will be more likely to rely on them.

The program is designed to increase your awareness of what affects your spine. When you watch your back, you will see how what you think, feel, and do has a direct effect on the health of your spine. Practicing the nine strategies of my program will help you to change the behaviors that promote back and neck pain and to replace those harmful habits with lifestyle choices that will reduce your pain. In the final chapter, I discuss complementary therapies, such as acupuncture, yoga, Pilates, and herbal remedies, you might want to explore to support your efforts to take care of your spine.

If all of this seems daunting, I want to reassure you that watching your back can become second nature, as it has for so many of my patients. I have learned that if a program is too demanding, my patients will not stick to it. Following the full daily routine takes less than fifty minutes a day. The good news is that the time is not consecutive. You do not have to carve out a big chunk of time at once. The workout takes only ten minutes, while the stretches take two or three minutes. Much of what you will be doing, such as posture correction stretches, deep breathing, and positivity practice, takes only two or three minutes a shot and can be done anywhere. Though I suggest a schedule, you can do these simple things at any time during the day.

You might want to ease into the program by focusing on one strategy that addresses your immediate needs. If you are under a lot of stress, you might want to start with deep breathing and mindful meditation. If your neck and shoulders ache from working at a computer all day, see what targeted stretches will do to ease the tension in your muscles and relieve your pain. Maybe your back pain is making it hard for you to get a good night's sleep. Paying attention to your natural biorhythms and changing your bedtime rituals could soon have you sleeping like a baby. You get the idea. Once a single strategy begins working for you, you will want to try another. The nine strategies complement each other, and their effects are cumulative. I do not want you to feel overwhelmed. Changing your life takes commitment. You have to embrace the strategies at your own pace. With consistency, watching your back will become automatic. The positive results of your attention will encourage you to do more.

The Watch Your Back program is incremental. You can expand or intensify what you are doing as your commitment grows. Nothing sustains enthusiasm for the program more than good results. When your aches and pains diminish or vanish completely, you will make the nine strategies a way of life because of their power to help you overcome your back problems. I know this from experience. I have seen how enthusiastic my patients are about the effects of their new routine.

SAY GOODBYE TO PAINKILLERS

Jennifer, an aide at a center for autism in her late twenties, suffered a back injury while working with a 200-pound disabled student who did not know his own strength. She injured her back so severely she needed to have surgery to repair it. Frustrated and depressed, she came to see me after an unsuccessful spinal fusion procedure. Her debilitating pain remained. Unable to do basic daily tasks, she had to rely on her husband to do everything, from taking care of her personal grooming to doing housework. She lay in bed, unable to move. Her weight started to go up, which made her even more miserable.

Before seeing me, she consulted with a series of doctors who prescribed a cocktail of prescription drugs, including Vicodin and muscle relaxers, which are routine treatment for her condition. In fact, patients with chronic pain account for 70 percent of the opioids prescribed in the United States.

Before long, she developed an opioid dependence. The drugs did not help her. She was functionally worse, barely able to move. When she began to mix drugs with alcohol, she knew she had to stop the runaway train she was on.

She went to her doctor's office with a grocery bag full of medication and a jug-sized bottle of vodka and told him that she was done with both. She then tried to manage her pain on her own without success.

She came to see me at New York Spine Surgery and Rehabilitation Medicine. She had heard that I believe in treating the whole patient. I introduced her to the Watch Your Back program. Seeing that she was significantly overweight, the very first goal was to help her take realistic steps to lose thirty pounds. She was carrying the extra weight around her middle. Her waist measured thirty-six inches, which meant the weight was putting more than forty-one pounds of added force on her spine. To put this in perspective, forty pounds is equivalent to four gallons of paint, a medium size bag of dog food, an SUV tire, or a fifteen-foot canoe. Imagine the spine experiencing that much additional force.

I encouraged her to lose one or two pounds a week to meet her goal in six months to a year. She began to eat a pain-killing, anti-inflammatory diet and her weight began to drop. She became more active, taking short walks and doing yoga. She reached her weight goal by year's end.

The results were life changing. The improvements she experienced made it easy for her to achieve a positive outlook on life and gave her confidence in her power to manage her pain. Then we were able to adopt some other aspects of the Watch Your Back program: I advised her to be mindful of the right way to bend, lift, twist, and reach at work to diminish the stresses on her spine. We created a program to get her moving, which involved walking, swimming, and riding a stationary bike.

In time, I was able to adjust her medication so that she could manage her pain without opioids. She was soon back on track without narcotics and able to resume her studies to become a behavior therapist.

Just like Jennifer, my patients have successfully incorporated the program's strategies into their daily lives without too much trouble. From a middle school girl whose heavy backpack strained her spine to a business man whose long international flights and carb-loaded eating while traveling took a toll on his spinal health; from a young mother whose back problems began when she was pregnant and intensified as she lifted and balanced her growing baby on her hip to a postal worker who moved heavy packages all day long, these are just a few examples of patients who have benefited from watching their backs.

I want you to become a success story, too.

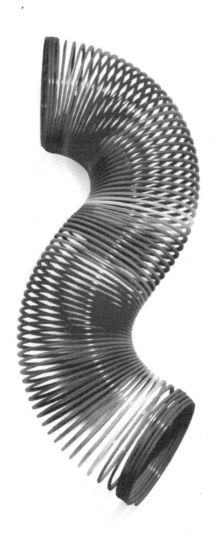

Part 1

What You
Need to
Know about
Back and
Neck Pain

Chapter 1

My Aching Back

My patients use so many vivid words to describe their back pain. On the spectrum from mild to severe, they report sensations that are: achy, burning, stabbing, stinging, shooting, throbbing, tingling, sharp, dull, constant, deep, well-defined, vague, annoying, gnawing, debilitating, all-consuming, nauseating, persistent, agonizing, numbing, stiffening, crippling, excruciating. People experience pain in very different ways.

The onset of back pain varies as well. Back pain can come in a flash or develop slowly over time. The pain may come and go or remain constant. Repetitive motions can result in pain that develops slowly and intensifies with time. Disc disease can produce flare-ups now and then, which can become increasingly severe. An injury from lifting something heavy, twisting, or bending the wrong way, or a sudden, jarring movement can cause immediate, acute pain. Sometimes pain develops or worsens hours or days after an accident or injury.

Pain limits people in countless ways. People want to be able to pick up their grandchildren, play a set of tennis, plant a perennial bed, or dance the night away. When pain makes it difficult to do even everyday things, such as tying their shoes, carrying groceries, or throwing a ball for their dog to fetch, the joy can seem to fade from life. The emotional component of pain, especially relentless chronic pain, cannot be underestimated. The sense of restriction can be very demoralizing. It can be difficult to focus on anything else but the pain, which only exacerbates the suffering.

The labels "acute" and "chronic" refer to how pain begins and how long it lasts. Acute back pain is often caused by an identifiable injury. The sudden, severe pain can resolve in a matter of days but may last up to six weeks. The intensity of a first acute episode can be so intense that people immediately seek medical advice. Over time, my patients learn how to deal with acute attacks as you will in the pages that follow. Instead of a sudden shock of pain that can make you want to lie flat on your back, chronic pain tends to develop gradually over time, but it can become progressively worse. Pain is considered chronic if it lasts at least three months or occurs intermittently over a period of six months. Chronic pain does not always have an identifiable cause.

Being in constant pain without knowing why can destroy the quality of your life. I have witnessed this tragic outcome far too frequently. When pain limits your ability to enjoy the things that give you pleasure, such as driving long distances to visit friends and family, playing soccer in a local league, or even thinking about sitting in a movie seat for a long film, a sense of deprivation can take over, which can lead to frustration and low spirits. The fear of making the pain worse can cause you to further limit your activities, and that will only intensify your distress. I have seen all too often that chronic back pain has a significant emotional effect on my patients.

What I see in my practice has led me to emphasize the psychological effects of back problems and to find ways to treat the mind as well as the body. I want to put you in control of your pain instead of allowing your pain to control you. The Watch Your Back program addresses the emotional and psychological issues that can feed your pain and prevent your healing.

I focus on this emotional component to help patients cope with and reduce their pain, as you will learn in the Watch Your Back program. To help you identify your back pain and deal with it, a closer examination of acute and chronic pain is in order.

ACUTE BACK PAIN

Acute back pain, which comes on suddenly, tends to be severe and short term. An acute episode lasts from a few days to six weeks. Most acute back pain is due to muscle injury, a strain or a sprain in the soft tissues supporting the lower spine or neck. Heavy lifting and repetitive motions can put too much stress on your back or neck muscles. The muscle fibers are stretched too far, and they tear. When these soft tissues are injured, your body springs into action to repair the damage by generating an inflammation response, the mechanics of which I will cover in detail in chapter 3. Inflammation causes the damaged tissues to swell, which results in pain. The affected muscles can go into spasm or become stiff. The pain can radiate from your spine to your buttocks, thighs, or knees. Sometimes people do not realize that a back injury or problem is the source of pain they feel in their knee. Properly handled, most, if not all, of the pain goes away.

The bad news is that 20 percent of those who experience the agony of acute back pain develop chronic pain with persistent symptoms that last a year. For some, back pain becomes permanent and disabling. Committing to the Watch Your Back program after you calm an acute episode will help you to avoid that fate and escape chronic back pain.

WHEN TO SEE A DOCTOR

The severe pain of an acute episode can be alarming. Many people immediately see a doctor for diagnosis and advice. Though the severity of an acute attack can be worrying, severe pain is not always an indication that something is seriously wrong. Acute back pain usually resolves on its own. After the initial episode, most people learn to wait it out. The fact is that back pain rarely requires urgent medical attention. You need to consult your doctor if:

- A child complains of back pain
- You have progressively worsening pain or weakness in your legs
- The pain is relentless or intensifies
- The pain disturbs your sleep
- You cannot stand upright

- You have a fever
- You are nauseated
- You lose bladder or bowel control

If you should experience any of these symptoms, I recommend that you seek medical advice.

ACUTE ATTACK: AVOID BENDING, LIFTING, TWISTING, AND REACHING

An acute episode of back pain is intense and hard to forget. You may have been laid low by the flash of sharp pain you experience when your back "goes out," to use a common expression. Some people take to their bed to rest their body. Though moving may be the last thing on your mind, extended bed rest is not the solution. A study found that patients who stopped everything to recuperate experienced more pain and made a slower recovery than patients who simply modified their activities. After a brief rest, remaining active, while careful to avoid physical activity that can trigger or intensify your back pain, will speed your recovery. By gradually increasing your physical limits, you will boost the circulation necessary for healing and release endorphins, your body's natural painkillers.

WHAT TO DO WHEN YOUR BACK "GOES OUT"

If you feel a flash of pain and think you have thrown out your back, stop what you are doing. Stand up and stand still. Do not try to push through the pain. Find a chair and sit upright to see if the pain subsides or diminishes. Try a few very gentle seated stretches (see pages 145 to 151) to see if you can relax your spasming or stiff back. If a stretch is painful, stop doing it. Lie down on your back, on the floor or your bed.

When in acute pain, you should avoid:

- Serious bending
- Lifting more than five pounds
- Twisting
- Reaching

In the first day or two, your objective is to reduce pain and muscle spasms. Rest and ice packs are your first treatments.

- If you feel incapacitated, try limited bed rest. By limited, I mean no more than two days of inactivity. Strong evidence shows that people who continue their activities without bed rest at the onset of back pain appeared to maintain better back flexibility than those who rested in bed for a week. Other studies suggest that bed rest may worsen back pain and can lead to secondary complications such as depression, decreased muscle tone, and blood clots in the legs.

- For the first two days, use cloth-covered ice packs in short intervals multiple times a day. Applying cloth-covered ice or cold packs to the location of the pain will reduce inflammation and ease soreness. The cold treatment will help to constrict the blood vessels, reduce swelling, and have a numbing effect. Ice presses can help to minimize potential tissue damage by slowing the flow of blood to the inflamed area. If you do not have a cold pack, a bag of frozen vegetables or ice cubes wrapped in a towel will work.

- Sleep and rest on your back to support the affected muscles. Use special pillows or lower back supports to take pressure off your back. No lumbar pillow? Make one by rolling up a towel and placing it behind the curve of your lower back. Avoid sleeping on your stomach, which can make your back pain worse.

- Taking an over-the-counter nonsteroidal anti-inflammatory drug (NSAID) such as ibuprofen (Motrin or Advil) or naproxen

(Aleve) can reduce pain and swelling. Only use this medication for a short period of time because NSAIDs can cause stomach and gastrointestinal discomfort and increase the risk for heart attack and stroke in some people. You can also take acetaminophen (Tylenol), which is less effective but easier on the stomach. Dosages should be discussed with your physician.

After two days, return to a near normal schedule to promote a rapid recovery.

- Ease back into exercise. Begin with gentle stretching. Build up to more rigorous movement and strength exercises.

- Introduce heat therapy once the inflammation has subsided. Applying heat for short intervals improves the flexibility of soft tissues, movement of muscles, and overall functioning of the back. Localized warmth stimulates blood circulation in your back, which brings healing nutrients to the injured tissues. If you do not have a commercial heat wrap, you can make a heat pack by filling a sock with rice and nuking it in the microwave. There are always old-fashioned hot water bottles. Even more basic, you can take a hot shower or bath.

Using this two-phase approach, most people experience a full recovery within two weeks.

ACUTE ATTACK

A forty-five-year-old computer engineer named Jack was caught up in a large project. He had spent twelve hours a day for weeks sitting in front of his computer. Jack stood up to go to a meeting one morning and felt a rip and a pop in his right lower back along with very sharp pain. He had such excruciating pain that he called for an immediate appointment. I was able to see him. His MRI and X-rays were all within normal limits.

One of the most common scenarios I see is a patient with acute pain on the right or left side of the lower back, which occurred with a click, snap, crackle, or pop. This pain is often caused by the dysfunction of the facet joints, the keystone of the spine. They provide motion in the same way hip and knee joints do. Athletes in particular need to warm up and provide a range of motion to their facet joints, which may be a source of power and flexibility in elite athletes. These joints need to move to stay functional, and are painful if they do not move. Special attention to the facet joints helps to prevent pain and suffering.

When people are sedentary and fail to provide the spine joints with range of motion, activities like getting up and down, walking, making the bed, or gardening become painful. The facet joints make up the roof of the canal where the nerve exits and have a nerve supply called the medial branch of the dorsal ramus. When the joints are dysfunctional, the nerve becomes painful. Any motion can cause the whole nerve, which exits underneath the joint on its way to the legs, to separately become inflamed and painful. When the sedentary person moves, sometimes the joint capsules tear and cause localized pain.

I treated Jack with a local injection of anti-inflammatories and Marcaine, a topical numbing medicine. I pressed down on his back at the site and gently moved the facet joint. He was 50 percent better immediately. I recommended light flexion and extension of the lower back, anti-inflammatories, heating pads, and long, hot showers. Within two weeks, he was back to normal.

CHRONIC BACK PAIN

If your back pain stretches beyond four to six weeks, the long-term suffering is labeled chronic back pain. Though it can be severe, chronic pain is more likely to be mild, nagging, aching, or burning and can be accompanied by numbness, tingling, stiffness, or weakness. Chronic pain is often related to the spinal joints, discs, or supporting muscles in the back. Stresses to bones, muscles, ligaments, joints, nerves, or the spinal cord may be involved. Disease and injuries are part of the picture as well. Pain can accompany any of these conditions. The nerve roots of the affected area of your back send signals through nerve endings, up the spinal cord, and into the brain where the signal registers as pain.

Often, the source of the pain is never identified. In the past, 85 to 90 percent of back pain sufferers never knew what was causing their chronic pain. Today, with physical examination, MRIs, and X-rays we are usually close to making a diagnosis. Most back pain sufferers never know what is causing their chronic pain. In many cases, the injury or condition that triggered the pain may be completely healed, but the pain persists. Though the original problem is unknown or has healed, chronic pain is real.

The biological mechanism behind chronic back pain is not completely understood. In the simplest terms, we believe that the nerve pathways that carry pain signals from the nerve endings through the spinal cord and to the brain may become sensitized. When these pathways are sensitized, you may perceive pain more frequently and more intensely. Even after an injury or disease has healed, sensitized pathways can continue to send signals to the brain. That pain can be worse than the pain produced by the original problem.

On a physical level, prolonged inactivity increases back pain because the spine becomes stiff, weak, and deconditioned. Physical movement and exercise stimulate the healing process for most back problems. Rather than bed rest and inactivity, controlled, incremental exercise often delivers the best long-term solution for healing your back, reducing pain, and preventing future problems. In addition to nourishing and repairing spinal structures, exercise will keep your back flexible and strong. At the same time, being active lifts your spirits by stimulating the production of endorphins, the "feel-good" chemicals produced by the central nervous system and the pituitary gland, that relieve pain and reduce stress.

Many studies have shown that limiting movement often leads to psychological distress, which in turn can amplify the experience of the pain. Chronic pain often goes beyond the physical.

A SLIPPERY SLOPE: PAINKILLERS AND BACK PROBLEMS

Jill is a sixty-three-year-old, retired social worker who suffered from chronic fatigue, anxiety, depression, and back pain. Jill had significant problems with performing everyday activities such as cooking, cleaning, and walking. She told me that she had accumulated many diagnoses over time. Her latest MRI of the brain showed early degenerative changes, which coincides with her forgetfulness. MRIs and X-rays of the lumbar and cervical spines showed degenerative changes without spinal compression.

Over time, she had been treated with five spinal surgeries of her neck and back. She had been consuming 100 mg of OxyContin a day for twenty-five years. Having just moved from New York, she was looking for a new spine specialist. She asked me to take over writing her narcotics prescriptions. She had been hearing and reading so much about OxyContin that she was eager to stop taking the drug.

I explained to Jill that after taking 100 mg of narcotics a day, a very large dose, for twenty-five years, she has consumed more than 500,000 mg of narcotics, which could certainly have led to developing a tolerance for the drug. I advised her that most opioids are metabolized in the liver by either the CYP2D6 or CYP3A4 enzyme systems. Aggressive in metabolizing narcotics, these systems alter the potency and medical effect of the drug. The patient is left requiring more and more narcotics.

I told Jill that chronic pain and depression are intertwined. Scientific studies of fibromyalgia, lupus, osteoarthritis, and rheumatoid arthritis show that people who experience more negative emotions also report more pain. These same people have higher rates of depression, back pain, and other mood problems. I recommended intensive psychotherapy for Jill. The psychiatrist treated her with talk therapy and anti-depressants. Her back pain lifted partially as her depression lifted.

One year later, Jill takes 80 mg of narcotics a day, prescribed by a chronic pain management specialist. She is now on NSAIDs, acetaminophen, and gabapentinoids, which are non-narcotic attempts to relieve her back pain. Anti-depressants prescribed by her psychiatrist have helped to lift her spirits. She claims her back pain is 25 percent better. Aqua therapy is her favorite treatment because she can exercise more without having to carry her weight in the water. Jill responded very well to acupuncture which helps her pain and improves her mood. She feels more grounded and calmer when she meditates.

Chronic back pain often leads to the long-term use of narcotics. Addiction to pain-killing drugs is a complex problem to eradicate. Multiple treatment options are necessary. The approach outlined in this story resulted in a happier patient, with less back pain, but she still required high-dose narcotics.

Dependence on narcotics has become epidemic. We doctors need to address treatment options early on by incorporating the strategies of the Watch Your Back program to reduce the need for painkillers. We can halt this cascade of opioid dependency or keep it from occurring in the first place.

THE CHRONIC BACK PAIN/ EMOTION CONNECTION

For many people, back pain emerges every so often, lasts a couple of days, and then goes away. Knowing that an end is in sight, most learn to deal with their pain. In contrast, chronic pain is relentless. Either there is no break from the pain, or it returns with regularity. I have seen how disruptive chronic back pain is in the lives of my patients. Pain can affect a patient's mood, concentration, memory, appetite, and sleep. For many, the mental stress caused by trying to cope with pain can seem as severe as the pain itself. What they are experiencing makes them depressed, anxious, and irritable. They feel out of control, and that mindset exacerbates their pain.

The fact is that the more difficulty you have dealing with stress, the more likely you are to experience pain. When you are in pain, you probably feel stressed and anxious. If you cannot handle the stress, your muscles tense up, which only escalates the pain you are feeling. A cycle of emotional and physical pain is set in motion.

Some people are so afraid of making their condition worse that they come to regard their back problem as disabling. Their fear leads them to construct mental barriers to physical activity. They doubt they are capable of activity and worry that too much movement could injure their back further and intensify their suffering. This avoidance of physical activity can easily become a self-fulfilling prophecy. It goes beyond not realizing the physical benefits of stretching and exercise. If you expect the worst, your pain will feel worse. That negative outlook can disrupt your brain chemistry and make your pain all-consuming.

At the onset of a back problem, the pain-sensitivity circuits in your brain are active. If the pain continues, the activity switches away from the pain circuits to circuits that process emotions. Pain is inextricably linked to emotions. That is why you are likely to become irritable and experience mood fluctuations when you are in pain. When your pain is chronic, physical and emotional pain can exist on almost the same circuitry of the central nervous system. The activation of complex brain systems may increase your awareness of pain and decrease your pain tolerance at the same time. That is a scenario you want to avoid.

Pain can rewire your brain. When you injure your back, the pain acts as a survival signal to the brain, which prepares your body for "fight-or-flight." In emergency mode, the brain changes physically and chemically in response to the perceived threat and sets off a cascade of changes in the body, including increased heart rate, increased blood flow to the muscles, and other stress responses, to prepare you either to escape the threat or to confront it. When pain is temporary, the body usually resolves these changes and returns to normal. Chronic pain prolongs these systemic and chemical brain changes, which can be physically harmful and lead to psychological changes. Over time, the changes affect the way your brain functions and result in changes in behavior.

Many studies have shown that there is a relationship between chronic back pain and mental health disorders. One study found that people with chronic back pain are more than twice as likely to experience depression, anxiety, substance abuse, and sleep deprivation than participants without back pain. Another study with more than 100,000 participants found that the relationship between chronic back pain and psychological and emotional disorders is bi-directional—a continuous loop.

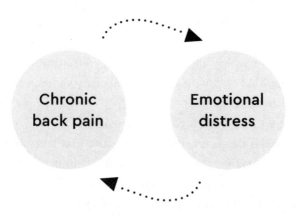

Chronic back pain

Emotional distress

To explain, the study showed that chronic back pain is a risk factor for depression, and depression is a risk factor for back pain. The participants with chronic back pain were six times more likely to be depressed than those who were pain free. Conversely, pain-free individuals who were subsequently diagnosed with depression were three times more likely to develop chronic back pain than those without depression. This study also found that the rate of depression increased with greater severity of pain. In short, chronic back pain can set off an emotional response that amplifies the pain, launching a cycle of physical and psychological suffering. Incorporating the nine strategies of the Watch Your Back program into your life is the most effective way to break that cycle or to prevent it from happening.

To give you insight into how everyday choices affect your back, the following chapter examines many of the common factors that contribute to back problems, most of which are under your control. Once you recognize the physical and mental triggers for your pain, you will be able to take steps to do something about it.

Chapter 2

Back Pain Triggers

Many factors contribute to back problems, and some of them might surprise you. Bad posture is a fundamental cause of back pain because it puts added pressure on the spine. When your posture is off, your spine has to absorb the stress. If your shoulders hunch and your head juts forward, the pressure increases wear and tear on the structures of your spine.

As you have learned, stress, both emotional and physical, set the stage for back problems. I do not have to tell you that jobs requiring heavy lifting, pushing, pulling, or repetitive movements raise the risk of injury and back pain. Improper movement while performing any one of these actions increases the likelihood that you will injure yourself.

You are probably aware that sitting at a desk bent over a computer all day or driving long distances without a break can be as harmful as physical labor. The "sitting disease" has become a well-covered health issue. A sedentary lifestyle can predispose you to low back pain, but all movement is not an antidote. High impact sports, like jogging, basketball, football, and soccer, or those that require twisting and turning, like tennis, golf, and skiing, can put stress on your spine, which can result in back problems.

Some physical attributes raise the odds of eventually developing an aching back. You are more likely to experience back pain if you are overweight, pregnant, tall, smoke, or have large breasts. Fashion can also take its toll on your back. Certain fashion statements can harm your spine over time. My goal is to raise your awareness of actions, choices, and attributes that are associated with back problems.

POSTURE—THE PRIMARY CAUSE OF BACK PAIN

Good posture is essential for spine health. Aside from improving your appearance, good posture will do you a world of good. When your body is properly aligned, your spine is supported by the right amount of muscle tension against gravity. Reducing stress on the ligaments that hold the spinal joints together helps to minimize the risk of injury. Good posture puts the least amount of strain on the muscles and ligaments that support your spine. With good posture, your muscles are more efficient, which prevents strain and fatigue. That translates to more energy.

I define good posture as ears aligned with the shoulders with the shoulder blades retracted or pulled closer together. A visualization exercise can help you to achieve perfect posture.

PERFECT POSTURE

Visualization can improve your posture. If you picture a straight line passing through your body from the ceiling to the floor, your ears, shoulders, hips, knees, and ankles should line up vertically.

To ensure good posture, imagine a cord is attached to the top of your head that is pulling you upward and making you taller. Do not allow your back to sway. Think of stretching your head to the ceiling without standing on tiptoe. Try to increase the space between your rib cage and pelvis.

Don't you feel better standing this way? Isn't it easier to breathe deeply?

Stop every now and then during the day and notice how you are holding yourself. If you find yourself slouching, remember this simple formula: ears aligned with shoulders, shoulder blades retracted.

The best sitting position depends on your height, the chair you are using, and what you are doing while sitting. The key to good sitting posture is feet flat on the floor, shoulders relaxed, back against the chair. Use a cushion or backrest to support your lower back if it does not meet the chair. Crossing your legs, slouching to one side, or slouching with your butt forward on the chair with a curved spine are bad for your back. You should avoid sitting slumped to one side.

The effects of good posture go beyond the physical. Research has shown a connection between poor posture and fatigue. One study found that patients with mild to moderate depression felt more alert and less anxious when they kept their backs and shoulders upright while sitting. Another study found that participants who slouched when they walked felt more depressed than those with good posture. When the slouchers shifted to a more upright position, their outlook became more positive and their energy levels increased. Additional research has shown that good posture improves self-esteem and mood in participants who were not depressed. You already know that there is a relationship between chronic back pain and depression and anxiety. Realizing that good posture can boost your energy and heighten your mood should be enough to convince you to make the effort to stand up straight.

When you realize how great an effect the way you stand or sit has on your pain, achieving good posture should become a priority. The idea that you can relieve or prevent back pain just by standing taller is a great motivator. Chapter 4, "Straighten Up," provides you with posture correcting exercises for common posture mistakes.

STRESS AND BACK AND NECK PAIN

Stress is a given in modern life. If worries and pressure get to you, it will wear you down, not only emotionally, but also physically. As I explained in the previous chapter, when you get stressed out, your body shifts into high gear. Your heart pounds, and your breath gets quicker. Your muscles tighten. This tension often occurs in the neck, shoulders, and down the spine. Prolonged tension in these areas can lead to back pain.

A stressful situation, such as a tight deadline or money worries, can trigger the "fight-or-flight" response, a powerful series of changes in your body to help you survive or escape a threatening situation. By getting maximum energy to parts of the body that need it most to protect you from physical harm, the response triggers a cascade of hormones, including adrenaline and cortisol, and physiological changes to help you fight off the threat or flee to safety. When you have a fear or worry, your muscles tense, and your heart rate and blood pressure increase. Your breath speeds up to increase the volume of oxygen in your blood. Blood flow to the surface areas of the body is reduced to minimize potential bleeding, while flow to the muscles, brain, legs, and arms is increased to provide adequate energy in your muscles for a fight or running away. Your immune, digestive, and healing systems are suppressed so that the emergency need for energy is prioritized. The "fight-or-flight" response is awe-inspiring to me. The body's coordinated, instant response to a threat is remarkable in its speed and intricacy.

If you are chronically stressed out, your body can activate the "fight-or-flight" response in reaction to stressors that are not life-threatening, like work pressure, marital problems, traffic jams, or even forgetting something on your shopping list. Though your body is not reacting to a physical threat, your psychological stress repeatedly activates the emergency response. Being in emergency mode for extended periods of time produces lasting effects on your physical and psychological health. Researchers have found that chronic stress contributes to high blood pressure and causes brain changes that may contribute to anxiety, depression, and addiction. Elevation of cortisol, known as the stress hormone, can lead to loss of muscle mass and increased fat accumulation. None of these potential effects is good for your back.

Stress and Neck Pain

A survey published by Statista.com found that stress is the #1 perceived cause of neck and back pain. Tension in the neck can cause muscle pain and headaches. If your posture is poor, your neck muscles are strained even more. Chronic neck pain can cause fatigue, depression, and irritability, which only increases stress and pain.

Stress and Mid-Back Pain

Pain in your mid-back involves muscles that are affected by breathing, namely the chest and shoulder muscles. When you are stressed, your breathing patterns change, becoming quicker and shallower. Your shoulders hunch up. These changes cause tension and strain and consequently pain in your mid-back.

Stress and Low Back Pain

The lower half of your back muscles affect flexibility and posture. I have noticed that many of my patients become more sedentary during stressful times. They do not stretch to relieve their tight muscles, which is a recipe for low back pain. When you are swamped with work and spend hours at the computer or bingeing an entire season of a TV show you had missed, you can strain your spine and lower back muscles.

The relation of stress to back pain is another example of the mind/body connection. As you will see in part 2, the Watch Your Back program has several strategies to help you relax, stop worrying, and lighten up.

INACTIVITY AND BACK PAIN

Being sedentary and unfit increases your risk of developing persistent back pain. Sitting for long periods of time has broader consequences, which scientists refer to as the "sitting disease." Inactivity has been linked to obesity, diabetes, and a high risk of cardiovascular disease.

Being active does immeasurable good for you. To put it simply, movement is good for your back and overall health. If you are suffering with back pain, activity increases blood flow to the affected area, which reduces inflammation and muscle tension. Moving also keeps you flexible, preserves your balance, and improves your posture. Regular exercise blunts the harmful effects of stress on your body, increases circulation, improves your sleep, and builds muscle mass, all of which contribute to the health of your spine. Weight-bearing exercise will strengthen your bones as well.

When you are active, you will not only look and feel better, but you will also be more optimistic. Exercise helps to lift depression and anxiety and boosts your sense of well-being. With these benefits, making moderate exercise a habit, like brushing your teeth, is the way to go.

One of my main goals is to get you moving. The program will give you tips on how to painlessly add more activity in your life. The benefits of doing so are incalculable.

ADDITIONAL RISK FACTORS FOR DEVELOPING BACK PAIN

Several physical attributes can predispose you for developing back problems. Being overweight, having large breasts, pregnancy, and being tall affect your spine. In addition to everything else that makes smoking bad for you, it is a habit that can promote back pain. Though you may not give it much thought, the clothes and accessories you choose to wear can have a direct effect on your spine.

Obesity and the Spine

My latest study involves the correlation between obesity, particularly in the form of belly fat, with spinal problems. In the U.S., more than two-thirds of adults (220 million plus) are overweight or obese, and childhood obesity affects 13.7 million children. As of 2016, 1.9 billion adults were overweight or obese globally. People now know that obesity is bad for their health. Excess belly fat is associated with diabetes, heart conditions, and metabolic syndrome. Given the media coverage, the fact is hard to avoid. But few connect being overweight with back pain. The findings of my study of the extra stress that excess abdominal weight puts on the spine are eye-opening. The amount of stress generated by abdominal obesity is significant. As waist circumference increases, so does the amount of stress on the spine. The greater the load, the more spinal stress increases. The result is back pain. Given the obesity epidemic, it is no wonder so many are suffering from back problems.

Belly Fat Effect on the Spine

As you will see in the charts that follow, our study used the waist circumference of men and women to calculate the force belly fat exerts on the spine. The chart shows the pounds of extra stress various waist sizes exert. Seeing a number that indicates pounds of force may be too abstract to have much of an impact on you. I have included a column to illustrate common items that are equivalent to various amounts of force.

Male

For men, the magnitude of forces generated by abdominal fat to the lumbar spine ranged between 3 and 120 pounds in our measurements.

Waist Circumference	Pounds of Force	Approximate Equivalent
25 inches	2.8	Steam iron
30 inches	11.7	Gallon of paint
34 inches	22.12	Sledgehammer
36 inches	27.56	2-year-old toddler
40 inches	38.46	Small outboard motor
45 inches	52.08	$1,000 in quarters
50 inches	65.71	58 hardcover books
55 inches	79.33	4 tires

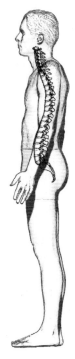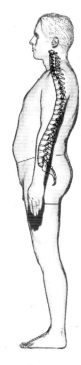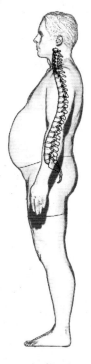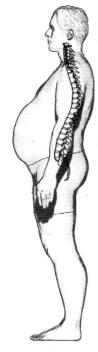

| 25 inch waist circumference 3 pounds force | 40 inch waist circumference 40 pounds force | 50 inch waist circumference 65 pounds force | 70 inch waist circumference 120 pounds force |

ABDOMINAL WEIGHT EFFECT ON THE SPINE IN MEN
Waist Circumference (Inches)

Women

The magnitude of forces generated by abdominal fat to the lumbar spine ranged between 5 and 170 pounds in our measurements.

Waist Circumference	Pounds of Force	Approximate Equivalent
25 inches	4.9	20 sticks of butter
28 inches	14.83	Pressure cooker
30 inches	22.2	2 bowling balls

32 inches	29.5	20 dozen eggs
34 inches	36.8	4 gallons paint
36 inches	44.2	Twin mattress
40 inches	58.81	9-year-old child
45 inches	77.13	16 bricks
50 inches	95.44	Baby crib
55 inches	113.76	60" flat screen TV

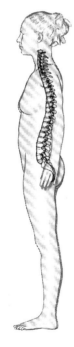 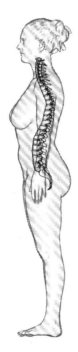 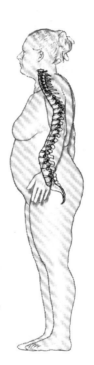 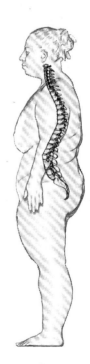

| 25 inch waist circumference 5 pounds force | 40 inch waist circumference 60 pounds force | 50 inch waist circumference 95 pounds force | 70 inch waist circumference 170 pounds force |

ABDOMINAL WEIGHT EFFECT ON THE SPINE IN WOMEN
Waist Circumference (Inches)

To put these numbers in perspective, you have to imagine what it feels like to lift this much weight. The magnitude of these forces is significant. If you are a man with a thirty-eight-inch waist, the excess fat in your abdominal area is equivalent to having nearly thirty pounds of pressure on your spine. For a woman, a thirty-six-inch waist is close to having forty-eight pounds of pressure on her spine. Imagine walking around all day carrying dumbbells that weighed nearly fifty pounds. That would be equivalent to carrying a large bag of dry dog food, six gallons of water, two cinder blocks, or, as the chart shows, a twin mattress. Not only would it be exhausting but carrying those weights would also cause major wear and tear on your back.

Your spine is designed to carry your body's weight. When you are overweight, your spine must assimilate the burden, which may lead to damage. The lower back is most vulnerable to the effects of obesity. In addition, abdominal fat interferes with good posture. Excess weight around the middle can alter the natural curve of the spine. The weight presses on the shock-absorbing discs between vertebrae, which can cause them to become dehydrated, herniated, or pinched, or create pressure on nerves that travel through the central canal. In addition, carrying extra weight can strain the muscles and ligaments that support your back, and you know what that means: pain.

Pregnancy

Back pain during pregnancy is a common complaint. As you gain weight, your center of gravity shifts forward as your uterus and baby grow. It is natural to compensate by leaning back to avoid falling forward. This change in posture can strain the muscles in your lower back.

At the same time, your hormones are relaxing the ligaments in the joints of your pelvis in preparation for the birthing process. This change may affect the support your back normally experiences.

It is especially important to be aware of your posture when you are pregnant. Stand up straight and tall and don't lock your knees. When you stand, use a comfortable, wide stance for the best support. If you must stand for long periods of time, take frequent breaks.

To avoid pitching farther forward when you are pregnant, wear low-heeled shoes with good arch support. Avoid high heels, which can shift your balance and cause you to fall. Some women find that wearing a maternity support belt is helpful, though not much research has been done on the subject.

A SHIFTING CENTER OF GRAVITY

Irene was a thirty-week pregnant patient from Africa who was suffering from severe sciatica. The obstetrics and gynecology doctor asked me to help care for her. Her pain was so intense that she was having difficulty walking. I researched and developed a plan for her that would allow any pregnant woman to keep her spine in optimal condition during the full term of her pregnancy.

I advised Irene that movement was necessary. Even taking short walks would help to reduce her pain. I instructed her to do a simple exercise while walking: to tighten her stomach muscles for a few seconds and then to relax them. I explained that doing this would help to strengthen her abdominal muscles, which provide stability to her lower back.

I did mention that she should trade in her high heels for comfortable shoes with good support. Wearing high heels can be risky for a pregnant woman because of the natural gravity shift with a growing belly and the added pressure on the lower back.

Next, I tackled posture. Maintaining good posture is especially important during pregnancy. Pregnant women tend to adjust their stance during the second trimester due to their shifting center of gravity. I suggested that she stand as straight as possible without leaning too far back or slouching to avoid placing too much pressure on her spine. She found standing up straight to be a problem as her pregnancy progressed. I suggested she might consider using a "sacroiliac belt," a supportive device used to stabilize the sacroiliac joint, to reduce pain in her pelvis and lower back.

Realizing that breathwork is critical in pregnancy, especially because of Lamaze techniques, I advised her to try deep belly breathing. Conscious deep breathing moves spinal nerves and joints and helps to keep the spine flexible.

Using more from the Watch Your Back program, I suggested she try mindful meditation to reduce stress and increase her sense of well-being. I explained that meditation would keep her centered and enhance her connection to her baby.

I asked her if she was having difficulty sleeping. She laughed and said she did not remember what getting a good night's sleep felt like. I suggested she try to sleep on her side, a position that would create the least pressure on her spine. I told her about special pregnancy pillows that would give her spine more support and eliminate additional strain on her spine while she slept.

We discussed her activity level before she was pregnant in order to design an exercise program that would work for her while she was pregnant. Adding to her walks, I suggested she try aquatic exercise, an excellent option for pregnant women because gravity is not an issue in water. Aquatic exercise does not place any unnecessary pressure on the spine.

Of course, stretching would relieve tension in her sore muscles. I gave her several stretches to do when she felt stiff or sore. I did advise her to be careful not to overstretch, which is easy for a pregnant woman to do because the hormone relaxin is produced during pregnancy to expand the uterus and soften connective tissue in the pelvis and the rest of the body.

I suggested she might want to try a prenatal yoga class. Some yoga poses help pregnant women and their babies to relax. I warned her that she needed to listen to her body, to never push into a position too hard, and to leave a pose gently. I recommended a few postures that are safe and effective for pregnant women: Seated Lateral Trunk Stretch (see page 146), Seated Forward Fold Stretch (see page 145), Seated Twist (see page 147), Cat-Cow Stretch (see page 169), Modified Downward Facing Dog (see page 148).

Irene appreciated my efforts to help her deal with her pregnancy-induced sciatica. She devoted herself to the program we developed for her. Her pain subsided, she delivered a robust baby boy, and mother and baby are doing well. Irene, sciatica free, is now enjoying a vibrant motherhood, and the bliss of her child.

Height

Being tall can be a predisposing factor for back pain. Your height might cause postural dysfunctions and muscle imbalances. If you are taller than everyone around you, you must often find yourself bending down to communicate with others. You may be forced to slouch at a computer. A desk chair that forces you to hold your head forward with your shoulders rounded is a formula for developing back pain. Sitting in such a position can overstretch your spinal ligaments and strain your discs.

Airplane, stadium, and theater seats are not designed for tall people. The legroom can be crippling. If possible, get an aisle seat. Cars, particularly back seats, can be a problem, too. Sitting in cramped quarters for long periods of time is not good for your spine.

Once again, good posture is the key to relieving your back pain.

Smoking

If you are still smoking, I have another reason for you to stop. Smoking increases the incidence of chronic pain. On one level, people who smoke tend to cough more. Coughing can injure your back, causing strained muscles or herniated discs.

Nicotine restricts blood flow to the discs in your spine that cushion your vertebrae. The reduction of blood flow can promote spinal degeneration. Though nicotine is a pain reliever, it acts as a vasoconstrictor, narrowing the blood vessels. When blood flow is reduced, healing is impaired because less oxygen is available. The spine is composed of bone, and bone needs a good supply of blood, water, and oxygen to stay healthy.

And speaking of bone, nicotine reduces calcium absorption, which prevents new bone growth. Smoking is directly associated with osteoporosis. When you smoke, your bones can become brittle and fragile and prone to fracture easily. With reduced calcium absorption, your bones will be slower to heal.

Large Breasts

The weight of large breasts can exert force on the spine, much as belly fat does. Large breasts can make good posture a challenge. Large breasts can make it difficult to stand up straight. Either leaning forward or hunching shoulders can throw the spine out of alignment. Of course, wearing a bra with good support is essential. Making the posture exercises and fixes (see pages 86–93) a regular habit will help with spine alignment and pain reduction.

THE PERILS OF FASHION

I am far from a fashion expert, but I know that certain fashion choices put your back in peril. Though there is nothing wrong with aspiring to high style, I want to raise your awareness of how your fashion choices can affect your back. There is so much variety in women's clothing, but many styles and fashion features can lead to pain as the following discussions demonstrate.

Heels

I would not dream of expecting women to give up high heels simply as a precaution. I understand why women are reluctant to stop wearing them. Stylish stilettos (or clogs, pumps, wedges—any kind of heel) not only add height, but they also make legs look shapelier. Many of my patients insist on wearing very high heels until their bodies rebel, and they no longer have a choice. At some point, their feet and back become so painful that they can barely hobble in their heels. Making a few adjustments can save your back and prolong your ability to wear high-fashion shoes.

Four-inch-high heels will do a number on your back if you wear them for long periods of time. Walking in high heels changes your stance. Your Achilles tendons, located in the back of your calves, become shorter and tighter. Repeated and extended wearing of high heels shortens the tendons permanently. When you choose to wear flat shoes, those tendons are forced to stretch, which may lead to inflammation and pain.

High heels tilt your pelvis forward, which deepens the curve in your lower spine, a position called lordosis. With a deeper curve in your lower back, your buttocks become more prominent and appear to be in a higher position. Your belly curves out. Though this curve in the buttocks and spine is considered attractive, it puts a strain on the nerves of your lower back.

I realize there is no way I can persuade some women not to wear heels, but there are many beautiful shoes with a reasonable heel height not higher than two inches. No more four-inch stilettos. If you must, limit your time wearing heels that high. Rather than wearing sky-high heels all day, save them for going out at night. You will be doing your back a favor.

Skinny Jeans

When you wear skinny jeans or "jeggings," your hips and legs are extremely restricted, which changes the way your body moves while you walk. You move in a restricted way that decreases shock absorption and adds stress on your joints, specifically your knees, hips, and lower spine.

You could consider wearing slightly looser-fitting jeans that are still form-fitting. Fashion does seem to be swinging that way. The best compromise is to refrain from wearing skinny jeans on days when you are planning to do a lot of walking.

Halter Tops

Regardless of how attractive they are, halter tops can pull your neck forward. This can add unnecessary strain to your upper back and shoulders. This is especially true if you have large breasts, which will put additional stress on your neck. In that case, wearing a supportive strapless bra will take the weight off your shoulders.

Pencil Skirts

Pencil skirts are popular because they are so flattering. The problem is that the cut of the skirt brings your knees in close and makes proper movement difficult. When you bend or walk, a pencil skirt can cause an unnatural strain on your hips and lower back. Over time, the strain can lead to painful disc or muscle problems.

Pencil skirts may be fine if you sit at a desk for hours at work, but you should opt to wear something else on days you expect to be more active. Another remedy is to wear pencil skirts with elasticity in the fabric to allow for more natural movements.

Shapewear

When buying support underwear, women often make the mistake of choosing a size that is too small. They assume that the tighter the shapewear, the better the slimming benefit. That assumption is a recipe for discomfort and eventually for back pain. Shapewear that is too tight restricts movement and creates additional pressure on the spine. To save your back, avoid squeezing yourself into a smaller size. Instead, buy shapewear in your actual size.

Heavy Necklaces

Wearing a "statement" necklace can have the same effect as halter tops. A heavy necklace can push your head forward, which increases the weight that your upper back and shoulders need to support. If that accessory makes the outfit and you are not ready to give it up, try to wear the necklace for special occasions only and limit the amount of time that you do.

Shoulder Bags

Shoulder bags are popular because they keep your hands free, but there is a downside. Slinging a bag over your shoulder creates an uneven distribution of weight on your spine. Always wearing your bag on the same shoulder can lead to muscle and joint asymmetry, which can become painful.

One solution is to pack your bag as lightly as you can. Another is to alternate shoulders when you carry a purse with one strap. If the strap is long enough, you can wear the bag across your body—with the bag on one side of your body and the strap looped over the opposite shoulder. A cross-body bag distributes the weight on both sides of your body.

A fanny pack is another option. With major designers including them in their lines, fanny packs are back in style. The bags are small and held very close to the body, which puts less stress on the joints of the spine and postural muscles. A fanny pack can prevent one side of your body from getting tense from doing all the work. You can avoid muscle spasms that shoulder bags can produce. Even so, make sure to keep the fanny pack as light as possible to keep from straining your lower back.

Heavy Bags and Briefcases

Carrying a heavy bag or briefcase can affect your posture. The weight of the bag may cause you to lean to the side. Routinely tilting your spine in that way affects the alignment of the spine and the compression can damage your discs, muscles, and ligaments.

Over-stuffing your bag or briefcase has multiple consequences because spine forces are a multiple of the weight of an item. The force of an extra book in your backpack may equal the force of the weight of seven books to your spine.

Avoid bags with thin straps or handles. Wide straps allow the load to be spread out more evenly across many muscles. This distribution of weight will lighten the burden on your spine and neck. Thin straps on heavy bags can cut deeper into your muscles, which can cause issues with blood flow.

Try to reduce the weight of your bag by eliminating clutter and non-essential items. If you carry a laptop and chargers for various electronic devices in your briefcase along with your work, you might want to balance the weight by carrying two briefcases. Many use a backpack, but you have to be mindful that the backpack is not too heavy. If you cannot avoid a heavy load, try using a small suitcase with wheels or a cart.

Backpacks

People of all ages, especially students, athletes, and members of the military, use backpacks. When a backpack is too heavy, people tend to lean forward to carry the weight. Leaning forward just twenty degrees significantly increases the stress on your spine.

People often sling a backpack over a shoulder using only one strap. Carrying a heavy backpack using both straps still exerts pressure on the spine and both shoulders, but at least the weight is more evenly distributed. Whenever you use a backpack, you should be sure to use both straps.

The rule of thumb is that you should not carry more than 10 percent of your weight in a backpack. If you weigh 140 pounds, the most your backpack should weigh is fourteen pounds. I am seeing more and more children experiencing back pain. Carrying textbooks, notebooks, school supplies, and lunch in a backpack can easily exceed the weight limit. My advice is for students to use wheelies to avoid back strain. There is no reason for anyone to be a beast of burden today.

LIGHTEN THE LOAD

Isabella, a fifteen-year-old, complained of having back pain, especially when she bent backward. Sports, carrying a backpack, or lifting just about anything caused pain. She was planning a backpacking trip that summer for which she would need to carry a forty-pound backpack. MRI and X-ray workups showed a normal spine with a slight increased curve in the upper back, called kyphosis.

I devised a six-month plan for her to prepare her body for the challenge. I worked with a physical therapist to teach her the principles of proper posture and to strengthen her spine. Her physical therapist trained her in good posture positions for her spine and pelvis. In addition, the PT taught her mobilization techniques for the facet joints in her spine.

She practiced flexion, extension, and side bending to move the facet joints. Our goal was to provide short-term pain relief and to restore pain-free motion by improving the range of motion of her spine.

She learned pelvic stabilization, which strengthens the muscles of the lower back and pelvis. These muscles support the spine and reduce the stress on the vertebrae of the lower back, which bears some of the body's weight. When Isabella achieved a full range of motion of the spine, she began strengthening the core muscles of her spine and abdomen.

Within six months, she was significantly more flexible and more muscular. I told her about my study about the forces that backpacks put on the spine. I explained that when a person carries forty pounds in a backpack, the spine force is seven times the weight or 280 pounds of force with good posture, and twelve times the weight or 480 pounds of force when leaning forward twenty degrees. I encouraged her to pack strategically for her trip by using lightweight materials and packing only what was necessary.

Isabella had a great trip. With her newfound range of motion and strengthened spine, she was able to enjoy a full day of backpacking and hiking. She knew not to push it and asked her friends for help when she needed it.

Back in school, she understands that she needs to strap her backpack correctly on both shoulders, maintain a good posture, and reduce the weight of her backpack by carrying some of her books in her hands.

Utility Tool Belts

Wearing a tool belt around your waist or hips may be efficient and helpful. The belt allows you to have what you need to do a job and leaves both your hands free. But tool belts can weigh fifty pounds when fully loaded. The weight of a tool belt puts significant strain on your lower back and hips.

Wearing a tool belt for an extended period can cause fatigue, discomfort, and severe lower back pain.

To prevent pain and strain, you can use a mobile toolbox or bucket-style tool bag instead of a tool belt. There is a new generation of tool belts designed to protect you from back pain. Many are padded and have suspenders to distribute the weight evenly between the shoulders and waist. When you wear a belt, arrange the tools so that the weight is evenly distributed. And of course, try to remove tools that are not necessary for the work at hand.

Knowing what can trigger your back pain is the first step toward preventing it from happening again. The next step is a quick anatomy lesson and a look at the physical reality of back problems.

Chapter 3

The Architecture and Lifespan of the Spine

B
eing able to visualize your spine and to know how it functions will help you to understand why the strategies of the Watch Your Back program work. This chapter is designed to give you a picture of the phenomenal structure of the spine as well as what can happen when your spine's health is compromised.

People tend to forget that the spine along with the brain make up the central nervous system. Both are so important that they are shielded. The skull protects the brain, just as the spinal column protects the spinal cord. The communication between the brain and the spinal cord controls everything your body does. The brain directs all the activity of your body through the spinal cord, which carries messages from the brain to the rest of the body. Consider the process a relay system.

Movement originates from your spine, which has three main functions:

- To protect the spinal cord and spinal nerve roots
- To provide structural support and balance for maintaining an upright posture
- To enable flexible motion

Without a healthy spine, everyday movement becomes difficult and painful. Imagine what life would be like if you were unable to sit up straight, bend over, pick up things, walk, twist, or turn your head. Such limited mobility is hard to imagine. It is easy to take movement for granted.

Your spine is at the core of your well-being, which is why it is so important to watch your back. A properly aligned spine is responsible for your flexibility and mobility. Even more important, when the alignment of your spine is off, your brain/body connection is disrupted. The breakdown in communication affects the way your body functions. When your spine is not healthy, you can develop hormone imbalances, migraines, mood changes, lower energy, sleep disturbances, a heightened sensitivity to stress, and more.

THE TOWER OF POWER

Your spinal column is a mechanical marvel comprised of thirty-three bones, called vertebrae, stacked on top of each other like building blocks—120 muscles, 100 joints, 220 ligaments, and 31 pairs of nerves all working together to help you stay upright and move. I like to think of the spine as the "backbone of well-being."

A brief introduction to the structure of the spinal column will give you a sense of how multi-functional your spine is. If your impulse is to skip the anatomy lesson, I promise there will be plenty of pictures. If you want to know what causes back pain, knowing what can go wrong physically is essential.

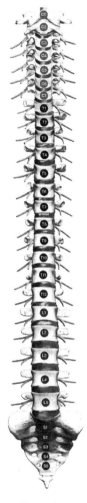
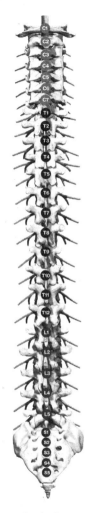
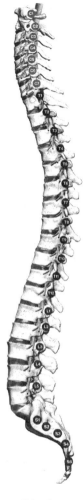

| Front view | Back view | Side view |

The spinal column is comprised of:

7   Cervical Vertebrae, called the neck

12 Thoracic Vertebrae, called the mid-back

5   Lumbar Vertebrae, called the lower back

1   Sacrum, called the tailbone

1   Coccyx, called the distal tailbone

There are five distinct spine segments that start at the neck and go down to the buttocks. The lateral view on the right shows the curves of the spinal column, which form an S.

Cervical (neck): The top part of the spine has seven vertebrae (C1 to C7). The neck vertebrae allow you to turn, nod, and tilt your head. The neck has an inward or concave shape, called a lordotic curve. The cervical spine is associated with the diaphragm (breathing), shoulders, parts of the arms, the esophagus, and part of the chest.

Thoracic (middle back): The chest or thoracic part of the spine has twelve vertebrae (T1 to T12). Your ribs attach to the thoracic spine, which makes this section of the spine less flexible. The nerves in your middle back communicate with parts of the arm and esophagus, trachea, heart, lungs, liver, gallbladder, and small intestine. This section of the spine bends out slightly in a convex, kyphotic curve.

Lumbar (lower back): Five vertebrae (L1 to L5) make up the lower part of the spine. The lumbar spine supports the upper parts of the spine. Connected to the pelvis, the lower back bears most of your body's weight as well as the stress of lifting and carrying things. That burden is the reason the lower back is often a hotbed of back pain. The lumbar spine bends inward, creating a concave, lordotic curve. The nerves in the lower back communicate with the legs and feet.

Sacrum: This triangular-shaped bone connects to the hips. The five sacral vertebrae (S1 to S5) fuse as a fetus develops in the womb. The fused vertebrae do not move. The sacrum and hip bones form a ring called the pelvic girdle. The nerves in the sacrum affect the bowel, bladder, and sexual function.

Coccyx (tailbone): Four fused vertebrae form a small piece of bone found at the bottom of the spine. Pelvic floor muscles and ligaments attach to the tailbone.

A CLOSE-UP

It is time to focus in for a close-up of the vertebrae. You need this picture to understand the diseases of the back, which I discuss later in this chapter.

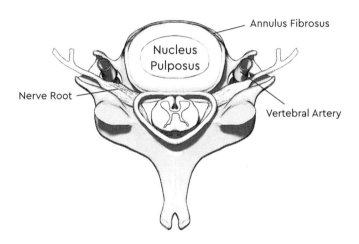

CERVICAL VERTEBRA—AXIAL VIEW

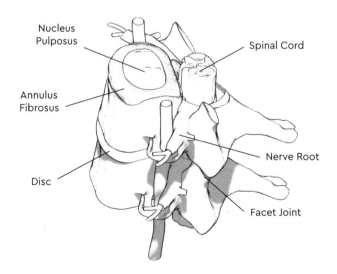

CERVICAL VERTEBRA—SIDE VIEW

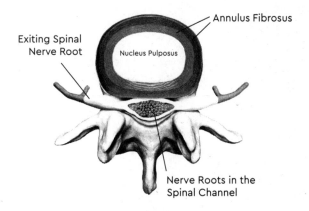

Exiting Spinal
Nerve Root

Annulus Fibrosus

Nucleus Pulposus

Nerve Roots in the
Spinal Channel

LUMBAR VERTEBRA—AXIAL VIEW

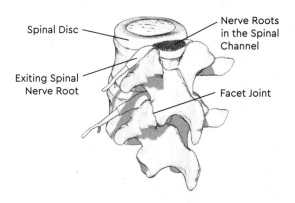

Spinal Disc

Nerve Roots
in the Spinal
Channel

Exiting Spinal
Nerve Root

Facet Joint

LUMBAR VERTEBRA—SIDE VIEW

The spinal column is a fortress to protect the spinal cord. A bony ring is attached to the body of each vertebra. When the vertebrae are stacked, the rings on each form a hollow tube through which the spinal cord passes. The spinal cord must be protected. If the spinal cord is injured, signals from the brain might not reach the body and paralysis may ensue.

There are three layers of protection inside the spinal canal. The walls are covered with a protective membrane, or sheath, called laminae. In addition, meninges, three layers of protection, surround the cord to shield it. Finally, cerebral spinal fluid fills the canal to cushion the cord.

The spinal cord is a column of millions of nerve fibers that extends from the brain to the first lumbar vertebra. At the top of the second lumbar vertebra, the cord divides into several groups of fibers, forming nerves that go to the lower half of the body.

You can feel the spinous processes when you run your hand down a person's back. A spinous process is a bony projection off the back of each vertebra. The muscles and ligaments of the spine, which are involved in rotation and keeping the spine erect, attach to the spinous processes.

A transverse process is a small bony projection off the right and left side of each vertebra. Spinal muscles and ligaments as well as ribs in the thoracic spine attach to the two transverse processes of each vertebra. The muscles that attach to the transverse processes maintain posture and induce rotation and side-by-side bending of single vertebrae and the entire spine.

An intervertebral disc serves as a cushion between two vertebrae. The flat, round cushions act as shock absorbers between the vertebrae. The outside of the disc, the annulus, is a strong outer ring of fibers, which help to keep the disc's center intact. The center of a disc, the pulposus, is soft and jelly-like. Needless to say, discs can be a source of many back problems.

Each vertebra has two facet joints, one pair faces upward and the other downward. The facet joints interlock with the adjacent vertebrae, connecting vertebral bones. Cartilage between the facet joints protects them from rubbing against each other, bone on bone. The joints allow motion in the spine, specifically flexion (bending forward), extension (bending backward), and twisting motion. Ligaments hold the two sides of the facet joint together.

The neural foramen are openings on each side between two vertebrae from which a nerve root exits the spinal channel. These nerve roots send signals to and from the brain for the rest of the body. Nerve roots can be a trouble spot as well.

As I said in the introduction, the architecture of the spine is miraculous in my eyes. If you take care of your back, your spine will remain a tower of power, which is why I designed the Watch Your Back program. I want you to keep your back supple, so that you can move with ease even as you age. A supple spine is a source of vitality and freedom—freedom of movement and freedom from pain.

THE FOUNTAIN OF YOUTH

Neil, an entrepreneur, was obsessed with finding the healthiest way to live. His spinal problems had constricted his quality of life and ability to play tennis. I operated on his back with a spinal fusion for a painful spondylolisthesis at the L4-L5. As he recovered from surgery, he wanted to know how to prevent wear and tear on his spine. He knew that gravity plus everyday movement could result in the spine's degeneration, resulting in such conditions as herniated discs, spinal stenosis, dowager's hump, and compression fractures. He realized that he had to watch his back if he wanted to move well and to do the things he liked to do. He knew that he could not be passive, that keeping his spine healthy had to become a priority.

I shared with him my firm belief that the spine is the Fountain of Youth. I told him that no one could accurately predict how a spine will age, but steps could be taken to slow down the process. I advised Neil to get to know the anatomy of his spine and to work on keeping it flexible and strong. I introduced him to the Watch Your Back program. I told him that once my patients took care to watch their backs, they were able to delay spinal aging. I explained that he, too, could protect his spine by incorporating the nine strategies of the program into his life. To take care of his spine, he had to foster the vitality of his "Fountain of Youth." The strategies that would help him achieve lasting spinal health are simple: straighten up, take a deep breath, move correctly and often, stretch, eat well, get restorative sleep, embrace positivity, and meditate. I told him that adopting these strategies would be the most effective way to tap into the Fountain of Youth at the core of his body.

Neil was glad to have a plan to fight gravity and the erosion of time. He has become one of the greatest followers of the Watch Your Back program. One year after surgery, Neil is pain free, fully functional, able to spend time at work and play. He is now enjoying life back on the tennis court.

THE AGING SPINE

Back pain is more common with aging because time and the force of gravity generate changes in spinal anatomy that cause stiffness, soreness, and creaking. As you get older, the moving parts of your spine wear out. For example, the discs shrink in height. They become less effective as shock absorbers, which means more stress is distributed on bone, nerve roots, muscles, and ligaments. The effects of bad posture begin to shift the curves in the spine as well.

Though most people begin to have back pain sometime between their forties and sixties, the spine often starts showing wear and tear before any pain is felt. In one study, MRIs were done on people in their twenties with no back complaints. The MRIs of this group showed that degenerative change had already begun in 37 percent of the participants. The MRIs of asymptomatic people in their fifties showed that 80 percent of them had spinal degeneration. Your spine is going to age. It is inevitable. But it is in your power to slow down the process and avoid painful conditions by following my program.

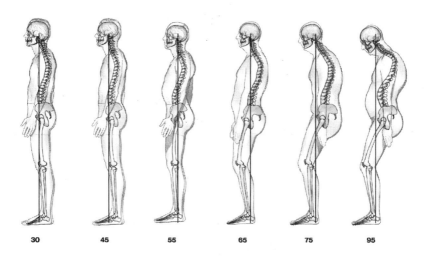

How the spine ages at 30, 45, 55, 65, 75, and 95.

No two spines are wholly alike, and some people have spine degeneration and herniations in their twenties, while others can maintain supple spines into their nineties. While spine degeneration occurs differently in all people, this process can be described. The following cascade is an account of general wear and tear based upon my observations of thousands of spine MRIs.

At thirty: Most spines typically show no wear and tear, and the curves show proper plumb line alignment. The plumb line, a line dropped from the top of the neck, is usually vertically aligned through the spine and body. The thoracic curvature is normal at twenty to forty degrees, and the lumbar curvature is normal at twenty to forty degrees. Hip and knee joints are flexible and show no stiffness. We see athletes engaged in sports for ten to fifteen years with early degeneration at the L4-L5 and the L5-S1. A herniated disc may be present in the neck or back at this young age.

At forty-five: Most spines are just beginning to show signs of aging. Injury and bad habits can speed up the aging process. The plumb line is usually vertically aligned through the spine and body.

At fifty-five: The spine tends to show some degeneration because of wear and tear to the disc space. Usually, posture is still good. The plumb line is usually vertically aligned through the spine and body. The average person may be primarily pain free, except for minor aches and pains. Smoking, obesity, a life of physical stress, especially bending, lifting, twisting, or reaching, or one of inactivity can lead to early degeneration. Disc problems can begin to occur. If your job requires you to sit for hours at a time or you have a sedentary lifestyle, your neck and shoulders could start to jut forward in middle age. Extended periods of sitting can shorten and tighten the hamstrings, which can lead to a contraction of the front muscles of the hip joint, called a flexion contracture. Both lead to a loss of flexibility.

At sixty-five: Degeneration is occurring at all levels of the spine. The neck can display increased degeneration. There may be the presence of spinal stenosis at C5-C6 and C6-C7, and the space around the spinal cord may narrow as arthritic ridges build up, contributing to that narrowing. The average person experiences aches and pains at sixty-five. Posture worsens as the neck and shoulders plunge farther forward—the plumb line shifts to the front of the body. The degeneration of the discs makes them thinner. This decrease in the volume and height of the discs can take inches off your height. When the spinal canal narrows in the lower spine, posture tends to tilt forward, opening the spinal canal and relieving the back and leg pain symptoms of spinal stenosis. The forward tilt flexes the hips, and the knee compensates by contracting. This makes the person shorter and stiffer.

At seventy-five: There is more wear and tear on the disc space. Arthritic ridges may build up further, leading to more severe narrowing of the spinal canal. The neck and shoulders plunge farther forward. The poor posture leads to significant aches and pains. Spondylolisthesis, a "slipped vertebra," is a condition in which a vertebra slips forward from the stack, tends to develop in the neck at C4-C5. The mid-back shows advanced degeneration with arthritis at T10-T11. The lower back shows progressive degeneration with a narrowing of the spinal canal at L3-L4 and L4-L5. Doing day-to-day activities can become impaired because of pain, loss of strength, and loss of balance. Osteoporosis, or bone loss, sets in, leading to collapses in bone height and compression fractures.

Further degeneration of the discs results in a person's losing more height. The forward tilt, caused by narrowing the spinal canal in the lower back, shifts the posture and plumb line once again. The vertical, or plumb line, is now positioned in front through the body. The hips and knees start to form permanent contractures. The person becomes shorter and stiffer.

At ninety: I am always so pleased to observe some of my patients in their nineties present with mild degeneration without spinal stenosis or fractures. Most others show advanced degeneration at all levels. The thoracic kyphosis curve may be more prominent with degeneration, and the compensating lumbar lordosis curve may also be more pronounced. A large S-shaped curve develops. There is more wear and tear on the disc space. Arthritic ridges may build up, leading to more severe narrowing of the spinal canal, which is called cervical stenosis in the neck and lumbar spinal stenosis in the lumbar spine. The neck and shoulders plunge farther forward. The poor posture leads to significant aches and pains.

The mid-back may show advanced degeneration. Women with osteoporosis may develop compression fractures most commonly at T10, T11, T12 in the thoracic spine or L1 and L2 in the lumbar spine. The lower back could show advanced degeneration with narrowing of the spinal canal at L3-L4 and L4-L5, called spinal stenosis. The forward tilt, caused by narrowing the spinal canal in the lower back, shifts the posture plumb line farther. The plumb line is now positioned well in front through the body. The hips and knees contract more, and the person becomes even stiffer and shorter.

Now you know why you tend to have more aches and pains as you get older. Being familiar with the geography of the spine will help you have a picture of the physical cause of some back problems. I have touched on the developing problems of the aging back in a general way in the preceding discussion. The balance of this chapter takes a closer look at the most common of these problems and diseases.

BACK ISSUES

Though you may never have a specific diagnosis for what is causing your pain, being familiar with what can go wrong with your back will help you discuss your acute or chronic back pain with your doctor.

Back Spasms

A back spasm is like having a charley horse in your back. A spasm is a painful and sustained contraction of a muscle. The sudden tightness and pain in one or more of your back muscles can be caused by an injury, such as a torn ligament, tendon, muscle damage, or a ruptured disc pressing on a nerve. Sleeping in an awkward position, bending, lifting, standing, or sitting the wrong way can be the reason your back is spasming. But the cause isn't always clear. You may never be able to identify why you experienced such sudden and intense pain.

Muscle spasms often occur when you are exerting a lot of energy or are straining, brought on by heavy lifting, working out, or a strenuous sports activity. If you are not sufficiently hydrated when doing any of these activities or your stores of potassium or calcium are low, you are especially prone to muscle spasms.

One theory to explain a spasm is that the body launches a protective response to an injury. The pain from the spasm immobilizes you, which prevents you from moving and making the injury worse. Another explanation for a back spasm is that the muscles are stimulated to brace the spine in reaction to something harmful or disruptive.

Strain and Sprain

A strain or sprain in the neck or back involves the soft tissue of the spine, which consists of ligaments, arteries, veins, muscles, and nerves. A sprain is an injury caused by stretching and tearing ligaments, while a strain is a similar injury to tendons. Ligaments connect bones to other bones, while tendons form a structure that connects muscles to bones. Ligaments tend to be more elastic than tendons. Ligaments are located at joints, and tendons provide the connection between muscles and bones that allows muscles to move different parts of the body.

Strains are common, especially for people who play sports. The damage happens to the tendon or the muscle to which it connects. Falling or twisting suddenly can cause a strain. People who are sedentary or have weak muscles due to inactivity are often more vulnerable to strains if they suddenly become active.

A strain can be very painful. A severe strain may take weeks or months to heal, but full recovery is typically the outcome.

Sprains can be a minor inconvenience or an injury that takes months to heal. There are three categories of sprains:

- Mild sprains involve stretching the fibers of a ligament without tearing.

- A moderate sprain occurs if the ligament tears partially.

- In the case of a severe sprain, the ligament completely tears, which makes the joint unstable. Severe sprains can require surgery.

Sciatica

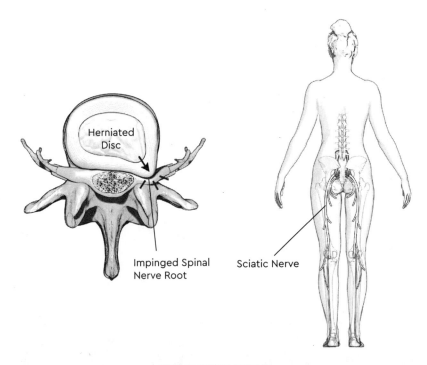

Herniated Disc

Impinged Spinal Nerve Root

Sciatic Nerve

THE SCIATIC NERVE

Sciatica refers to pain that radiates along the path of the sciatic nerve, which branches from your lower back through your hips and buttocks and down each leg. Typically, sciatica affects only one side of your body. You might feel discomfort almost anywhere along the nerve pathway, but the pain is usually from your lower back down to your thigh and calf.

When a torn disc, bone spur on the spine, or a narrowing of the spine compresses part of the sciatic nerve, inflammation occurs. Numbness, tingling, or weakness of the leg is the result. The pain varies from a mild ache to a sharp burning sensation to excruciating pain. Sciatica tends to affect people between the ages of thirty and fifty. Most people recover fully from sciatica, often without treatment. If you experience loss of feeling or weakness in the affected leg, check with your doctor immediately.

Osteoarthritis of the Spine

Arthritis in the spine occurs when the cartilage in the aligning facet joints erodes as a result of injury, wear and tear, or misuse. The facet joints may thicken and harden with age, causing a painful friction.

Proper movement will take stress and pressure off the joints in your spine, which can help you to avoid developing this condition or stop its progress.

Degenerative Disc Disease

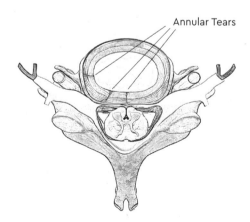

DEGENERATIVE DISC DISEASE OF THE NECK—AXIAL VIEW

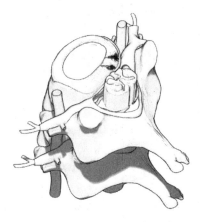

DEGENERATIVE DISC DISEASE OF THE NECK—SIDE VIEW

Degenerative disc disease in the neck is shown with the development of annular tears. These annular tears may spill inflammatory mediators, causing chemical irritation of the nerve roots and the spinal cord.

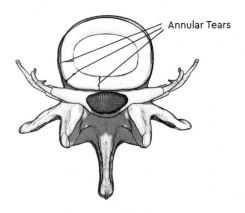

Annular Tears

DEGENERATIVE DISC DISEASE OF THE BACK—AXIAL VIEW

Early degenerative disc in the back with a process of tears in the annulus is shown here. With wear and tear, further annular damage occurs from time to time. These annular tears may spill inflammatory mediators, causing chemical irritation of the nerve roots.

Degenerative disc disease is not really a disease. The term refers to the effects of wear and tear on the disc, which occurs naturally with aging. Early degenerative disc disease manifests as tears in the annulus of the disc. Sometimes further wear and tear causes more damage to the outer layer of the disc.

A car accident, hard labor, and repetitive activities can produce traumatic degeneration regardless of a patient's age. Patients with degenerative disc disease in the neck usually complain of neck pain through the shoulder blade. Sitting or standing upright can exacerbate the pain because there is more pressure on the disc. My patients describe the pain as being deep, dull, and aching. The pain typically progresses from the neck into the shoulder, and in some cases the pain travels down the arm.

People with disc cartilage problems tend to have more pain when sitting and feel better when standing. Others have more back pain when they stand. The problem can be arthritis in the facet joints in the back of the spine. People who have this problem tend to hunch forward when walking. They feel better when they sit.

When degenerative disc disease occurs in the back the symptoms that patients report are a deep, dull, aching pain that is usually localized or travels to the buttocks, and in some cases the pain may travel down the legs.

The tears in the annulus fibrosus may set off an inflammatory response, which can irritate the nerve roots and the spinal cord. Later, the breakdown and the collapse of the facet joints causes mechanical pain. This is a deterioration of the back joints. The term radiculopathy refers to this irritation of the nerve root. When this happens, the symptoms are pain, numbness, and weakness in the zone of the nerve root.

Herniated Disc

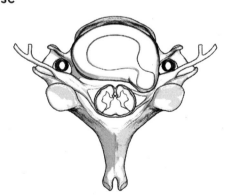

HERNIATED CERVICAL DISC WITH COMPRESSED NERVE—AXIAL VIEW
A herniated disc occurs when the nucleus pulposus exits through the annulus fibrosus. Notice how the exiting nerve is mechanically compressed and inflamed.

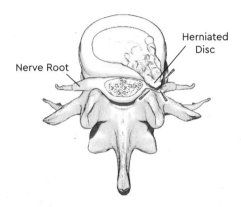

Herniated
Disc

Nerve Root

HERNIATED LUMBAR DISC WITH COMPRESSED NERVE—AXIAL VIEW

A lumbar disc herniation occurs when the nucleus pulposus exits through the annulus fibrosis. Notice that the nerve is mechanically compressed and inflamed.

If a disc is worn or injured, the pulposus, the soft gel in the center of the disc, may squeeze through the fibrous outer ring, the annulus. The rupture can occur between two vertebrae into the spinal canal or into the opening from which the nerve roots exit the vertebrae. The leaked pulposus may press on spinal nerves, causing pain. Though discs can herniate anywhere along the spine, they most often occur in the neck and lower back.

If a cervical disc herniates, the pain can increase when you bend or turn your neck. In addition to pain in the back or sides of your neck, a herniated disc in the neck may cause pain between your shoulder blades. The pain may travel to your shoulder, arm, hand, or fingers. You may experience weakness, numbness, or tingling in your arms.

If a disc herniates in the lower back, you might experience pain in your sciatic nerve. The sharp pain usually shoots down one side of your buttocks into your leg and sometimes your foot.

The pain from a herniated disc may go away in about a month as the disc heals. The at-home treatment is the same as the treatment for acute back pain (see page 12). Sometimes a herniated disc gets worse, especially if you repeat the activities that might have caused the rupture, for example, a job that requires heavy lifting. A worsening ruptured disc may cause chronic pain, weakness, or a loss of sensation in the affected area. If your symptoms get worse over time or you are not better after four to six weeks, see a doctor.

People ages thirty to fifty are most likely to develop a herniated disc. Following the Watch Your Back program will help you to avoid rupturing discs in your spine. Good posture, stretching, and regular exercise will keep your back strong and fit. Avoiding high heels and cigarettes will also help you avoid ruptures in your discs.

DISC REPAIR WITHOUT SURGERY

Frank, fifty-two years old, worked as a nurse on the night shift at the hospital. He complained to me of back pain that radiated down both legs, which was getting progressively worse. An MRI scan showed a small herniation at the L2-L3 and a large superiorly disc herniation at the L4-L5. I advised Frank that the L4-L5 needed to be decompressed in surgery.

Frank confided that he was terrified of surgery. He suffered panic attacks and could not even begin to think of having surgery. He asked me to help him as best I could without performing surgery.

For one of his flare-ups, I treated him conservatively with NSAIDs (non-steroidal anti-inflammatories) such as Advil or Aleve and gabapentin, a prescribed medication that stabilizes nerves. Because of the inherent drowsiness caused by the gabapentin, I prescribed it mainly at night.

I cautioned Frank to avoid bending, lifting, twisting, and reaching because these activities exert additional forces to the spine. I recommended that he add aerobic exercises, for example walking, swimming, or stationary biking, to his routine. Frank had been spending time in the gym doing circuit training. I advised him that squatting or deadlifting were not moves for him. Wall squatting (see page 152) with great care is usually tolerated well by patients. These forms of exercise produce forces on the spine that would be too much to bear, especially with his herniated L2-L3 and L4-L5 levels, where the spinal nerve roots are already compressed.

Physical therapy and core strengthening helped to improve his posture. Frank became stronger as he was rehabilitated. A chiropractor friend of his performed gentle manipulations of his spine.

Frank told me that he found the Seated Pigeon Stretch (see page 149) worked well to relieve his sciatica. Do not try this stretch if you have a hip replacement for fear of dislocation.

A recent follow-up MRI showed the disc at the L2-L3 was much smaller, and the large herniation of the disc at the L4-L5 had disappeared. Frank's pain came and went for the past five years, but it did not interfere with his life. He is careful and only experiences flare-ups from time to time. He knows how to handle those flare-ups. By staying fit, he is able to continue with the demanding physical work of nursing.

Spinal Stenosis

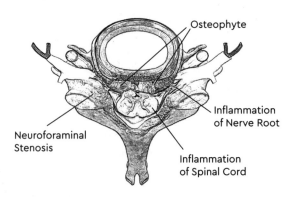

SPINAL STENOSIS OF THE NECK—AXIAL VIEW

An osteophyte, called a *bone spur*, is a bony or calcified hardening that could compress the spinal cord or nerve root. This image demonstrates compression of the spinal cord and the nerve roots in the neck. When the nerve root is compressed, it is called *neuroforaminal stenosis*.

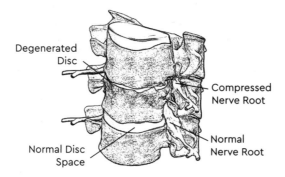

Degenerated Disc

Compressed Nerve Root

Normal Disc Space

Normal Nerve Root

SPINAL STENOSIS OF THE NECK—SIDE VIEW

Figure showing spinal stenosis arthritic buildup blocking the cervical spinal channel and compressing the spinal cord and exiting nerve roots.

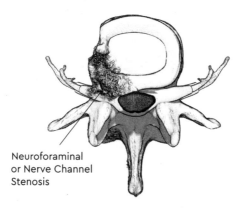

Neuroforaminal or Nerve Channel Stenosis

SPINAL STENOSIS OF THE BACK—AXIAL VIEW

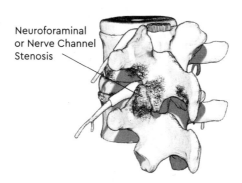

Neuroforaminal or Nerve Channel Stenosis

SPINAL STENOSIS OF THE BACK—SIDE VIEW

Figure showing lumbar spinal stenosis arthritic buildup blocking the spinal channel and impinging the root nerve.

The combination of spinal disc degeneration with arthritis in the joints of the spine can lead to a narrowing of the space around the spinal cord and/or nerve root, a condition known as spinal stenosis. The central channel carries the spinal cord and both nerve canals. Arthritis spurs may build up on the facet joints in the back of the spine due to activity, time, and wear and tear. The arthritic spurs begin to encroach on the nerve channels and pinch the nerve roots. This can happen anywhere on the spine.

Depending on what nerves are affected, stenosis may cause pain in the neck, shoulders, arms, and legs. When the spinal cord is compressed, a weakness or numbness in the legs and a shuffling gait may develop. You can lose coordination in one or both of your legs. Some of my patients have experienced lightning-like sensations down the back when they bend their neck forward.

When spinal stenosis occurs in the neck, my patients complain of:

- Numbness or tingling in a hand, arm, foot, or leg

- Weakness in a hand, arm, foot, or leg

- Problems with walking and balance

- Neck pain

- In severe cases, bowel or bladder dysfunction (urinary retention, or urgency and incontinence); if bowel or bladder dysfunction occurs, seek immediate medical attention

When spinal stenosis occurs in the lower back, symptoms include:

- Pain in the lower back

- Sciatic-type pain in the legs

- Pain on standing with relief from sitting or lying down

- Pain in calves when walking short distances

- Greater ease walking uphill than downhill

- The ability to ride a bike with ease

I have observed a symptom, which I call the "shopping cart sign." Patients with spinal stenosis report that they are able to walk long distances holding onto a shopping cart. Usually, they are stooped over, which opens the lumbar spinal channels. The same mechanics may be in effect with bike riding.

A doctor should monitor this condition.

Spondylolysis and Spondylolisthesis

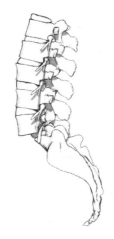

SPONDYLOLISTHESIS

Spondylolisthesis is a condition in which one vertebral body slips over another. It is predominantly a problem of the lumbar spine, although slippage of the vertebral body can occur in the neck.

Spondylolysis is a weakness or stress fracture in the facet joint area. This condition is a common cause of lower back pain in people under twenty-six, particularly athletes who put a lot of stress on their backs or overstretch their spines. High-impact activity can aggravate the condition.

With spondylolisthesis, a vertebra slips forward over the one below when ligaments loosen and discs collapse. When the facet joints become weak due to the degeneration of normally stabilizing structures, spondylolisthesis can occur. Aging, erosion, and trauma can cause spondylolisthesis. Degenerative disc disease and facet arthritis may occur simultaneously.

Patients who have developed spondylolisthesis complain of back pain and a dull pain from the buttocks to the back of the thigh. Many report hamstring tightness and spasms. Some patients have no symptoms. In advanced cases, the patient may have a swayback with a protruding stomach, a shortened torso, and a waddling gait.

Osteoporosis

Osteoporosis can take its toll on the aging spine. Nine million osteoporotic fractures, one every three seconds, occur annually worldwide. The condition causes bones to become weak and brittle. In fact, the term means porous bone. Bone is living tissue that is always being broken down and replaced. Osteoporosis occurs when bone breaks down faster than it can reform, which results in low bone density. You reach your peak bone mass by thirty. As you age, you lose bone mass faster than it is created. If you develop osteoporosis, your bones can become so brittle that a fall, bending over, or coughing can cause a fracture.

The condition is one of the most common causes of back pain in the United States. Osteoporosis can lead to compression fractures in the vertebrae. The condition can cause a vertebra to collapse over time. In the early stages of bone loss, there usually are no symptoms. When your bones have been progressively weakened, these symptoms may appear:

- Bones that break more easily than expected

- Back pain from a fractured or collapsed vertebra

- Loss of height over time

- A stooped posture, known as "dowager's hump"

A healthy diet, which includes calcium and vitamin D, and weight-bearing exercises help to prevent bone loss. Women over sixty-five years and men over seventy years require bone mineral testing with a DXA scan ordered by their doctors. Higher risk people with low body weight, smoking history, or a previous fracture may be tested younger.

BUILDS STRONG BONES

Sara, a sixty-four-year-old patient, became intent on taking care of her spinal health. Her mother had broken her hip and was forced to use a wheelchair in her final years. Sara suspected that her mother had osteoporosis and did not want to suffer the same fate. Hearing her concerns, I ordered a DXA scan, which measures bone strength and the risk of developing osteoporosis.

The scan showed that Sara suffered from osteopenia, a condition in which the body does not make new bone as quickly as it reabsorbs old bone. She did not have osteoporosis, a more extreme condition in which bone breaks down much faster than it builds up. The end result is fragile bones.

Osteoporosis is a silent disease. People often first discover they have it when they break a bone. Medically, such breaks are called fragility fractures, which appear in the vertebrae, ribs, hips, and wrists. A compression fracture of the spinal vertebrae may cause the affected vertebra to collapse from above or below. Most patients with vertebral fractures complain of back pain, usually sudden. In time, patients with this type of spinal fracture stoop forward as the vertebra loses height.

Sara wanted to know what she could do to strengthen her bones and protect her spine.

I told her that people reach their peak bone mass between the ages of twenty-five and thirty. By forty, bone mass declines slowly.

I explained to Sara that good posture was the best way to protect her spine, that when the spine is not in alignment, the forces on the spine increase. She understood that misalignment could lead to tons of pounds of forces on her spine each year. She began to see how poor posture would produce significant wear and tear on her spine.

I told Sara to put on her walking shoes and to walk more. A weight-bearing exercise, walking builds strong bones. The many additional benefits of walking include increased mental clarity, spine facet joint mobility, and nerve root mobility and function in the spine. I went on to explain that when she walks uphill her spine joints are in a flexed, open position, which may be helpful in conditions with root tightness. Uphill walking may even help patients with spinal stenosis because it opens up the spinal channel. When she walks downhill, her spine joints are in an extended, compressed position, which could worsen conditions involving nerve root tightness. The spinal canal tends to close with downhill walking. I suggested that strengthening exercises would stabilize and support her spine.

I advised Sara to consider safety to prevent fracture-causing accidents. Falls are the most significant risk factor. I told her that she had to be mindful of where she was going and to remove potential stumbling blocks at home to avoid falls that could fracture brittle bone.

The next step in protecting her spine involves nutrition. Great bones are made by paying attention to calcium and vitamin D intake. I worked with Sara to have her medical doctor check her blood tests and supplement her vitamin D levels. More than 50 percent of the world's population is vitamin D deficient. If you avoid the sun, have milk allergies, or follow a strict vegetarian or vegan diet, you might be at risk for vitamin D deficiency. Also, I recommended that Sara increase her calcium intake with foods, and she supplements the remaining amount of calcium to bring her into an optimum range based upon her age and medical needs.

Some say that precautions to prevent osteoporosis should begin as early as childhood. Sara was relieved when I told her that it was not too late for her, that medications are available to rebuild bones and to stop further bone loss. She left my office with a plan to save her spine.

It would be wonderful if we could diagnose the source of back pain every time, but most people never learn the cause of their suffering. Back pain often develops without a cause that your doctor is able to identify with a test or an imaging study. That is why the Watch Your Back program is so comprehensive. I saw the need for a daily routine that addresses the health of the entire spine and the recognized triggers for back pain, both physical and emotional.

Part 2 introduces you to the nine healing strategies of the Watch Your Back program. In each chapter, I explain why the strategy is effective and spell out what you need to do to incorporate the strategy into your daily life. Raising your awareness of how you stand, sit, and move, working to strengthen your spine and increase flexibility, eating a pain-reducing diet, getting enough restorative sleep, and de-stressing will go a long way to easing your back and neck pain. You have had an introduction to the spine and what could be the source of your pain. Now it is time for you to take action.

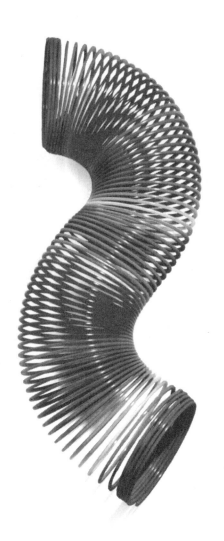

Part 2

How to
Watch Your
Back

Chapter 4

Strategy 1:
Straighten Up

n 2014, I released what became known as my "text neck" study. As a spine specialist, I could not help noticing that using smartphones and electronic devices was resulting in poor posture. People were bending their heads forward to read their screens. At the same time, more and more of my patients were complaining of neck and back pain. I realized there had to be a connection.

SCREEN TIME AND YOUR NECK

The case of one patient convinced me that text neck was becoming a health concern. This thirty-two-year-old patient worked in a warehouse as a supervisor. He developed a herniated disc, which caused persistent pain in his legs. Surgery successfully decompressed the affected disc. His leg pain went away.

Six weeks of light rehabilitation was necessary before he could return to work. He needed progressive strength training for another six weeks before he was doing full duty with the capability to lift. Before long, he developed back pain and neck pain. A new MRI showed that the surgery site was not the problem. We treated him with continued physical therapy.

One day, as we were trying to find the source of his pain, he admitted he was addicted to the video game Angry Birds, which he played on his cell phone about four hours a day.

When he played the game, he bent his head way down. He played with his phone a little below chest level. Looking down as he played, he bent his head more than 90 degrees. The ligaments and muscles in his neck had become inflamed because his tilted head was loading additional stress on his neck.

I explained how he could position his phone to avoid text neck by holding the screen at eye level. I recommended heads-up postural training with physical therapy to help to correct the problem. I advised him to be mindful of how he was standing and sitting and to do the posture correcting exercises from my program, along with the Watch Your Back workouts. His posture improved. In one month, he was pain free.

My research found that adults spend an average of two to four hours a day, teenagers decidedly more, with their heads tilted forward to read, text, game, and watch movies and shows on smartphones and devices. Cumulatively, this adds up to 700 to 1,400 hours a year of excess stress on the cervical spine. My study measured the dramatic increase in pressure on the spine when the head is flexed forward at varying degrees.

We were able to quantify the additional force produced by tilting the head. Standing or sitting with good posture, head held straight, produces ten to twelve pounds of force on the neck. At sixty degrees, the spine is subjected to sixty pounds of force. An article on the study, which appeared in *The Atlantic*, gave sobering equivalents for that sixty pounds. Tilting your head forward sixty degrees creates the pressure of carrying four bowling balls, six grocery bags full of food, or an eight-year-old child on your neck. Imagine the wear and tear that sixty pounds of force creates on the neck and spine. No wonder I had been seeing such an increase of neck and back pain complaints in my practice.

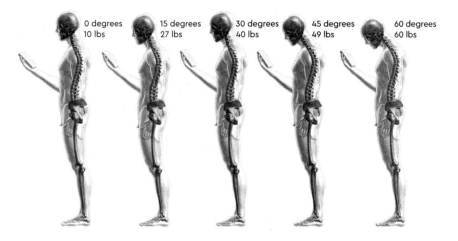

| 0 degrees | 15 degrees | 30 degrees | 45 degrees | 60 degrees |
| 10 lbs | 27 lbs | 40 lbs | 49 lbs | 60 lbs |

An adult head weighs 10 to 12 pounds in the neutral position. As the head tilts forward the forces on the neck surge, as shown.

The text neck study should open your eyes about the stresses and strains bad posture can create.

GOOD POSTURE: THE BENEFITS

In the broadest sense, good posture helps to develop flexibility, strength, and balance in your body. Good posture puts the least strain on muscles and ligaments while you are moving or sitting. This reduction of stress leads to less muscle pain, more energy, and lowers the risk of injury. Though the list of benefits for your entire body is impressive, standing and sitting correctly is the best way to save your spine and slow down degeneration. Good posture:

- Prevents backache and muscular pain.
- Keeps bones and joints in alignment, which ensures muscles are used properly.
- Reduces fatigue because the muscles are working efficiently and using less energy.
- Helps to reduce the wear and tear of joints.
- Prevents the onset of arthritis.

- Decreases the strain on spinal ligaments.

- Prevents the spine from becoming fixed in abnormal positions.

BAD POSTURE: THE NEGATIVE EFFECTS

Bad posture has an impact on your health in ways you might not think of. Not standing or sitting straight can negatively affect important bodily functions, including:

Circulation

Your body needs a continuous and healthy blood flow. Bad posture, particularly when sitting, constricts the flow of your blood and can cause blood to collect in the veins for long periods of time. Poor posture can contribute to high blood pressure because slouching can decrease blood flow to and from the heart. Poor circulation also leads to developing varicose veins.

Breathing

Slouching limits the capacity and function of your lungs. To breathe properly your diaphragm needs enough space in the thoracic cavity to release and contract with each breath. That space is compressed when you hunch forward. When your shoulders are rounded, it is more difficult to take a normal, deep breath. When your body is lengthened and in alignment, your ability to breathe is not impaired. You are able to inhale the oxygen you need to restore and rejuvenate all the cells in your body. Studies have shown that with good posture lung capacity can improve by 30 percent over time.

Digestion

If you sit slouching with your shoulders over your stomach and chest, you compress the organs in your abdomen. This slows digestion, which affects your metabolism and the way your body processes foods.

Sleep

The neck pain, back pain, and increased stress levels caused by bad posture can directly interfere with getting quality sleep. Lower back and neck pain are the result of small tears in muscles that occur during the day. The pain of overstressed back muscles can make it hard to relax. You might toss and turn to find the right position. Your posture can lead to insomnia, apnea, and other sleep problems.

A vicious cycle can be set in motion. Not getting enough sleep can make you more vulnerable to stress the following day. The rise in stress levels when you are sleep-deprived can create tension in your body that leads to slouching during the day.

If you do not get enough restful sleep, your muscles will not have enough time to repair during the night. The pain continues the following day, which leads to more sleeplessness. Studies have found that people with moderate-to-severe sleep problems are more likely to develop chronic pain after a year than those who sleep well.

Sex

Sloping sitting, also known as sacral sitting, is the culprit here. This posture involves leaning back with your bottom at the edge of the seat. This position shortens and tightens the pelvic floor muscles, which are the primary sex muscles. When these muscles are tight, they cannot exert power. The result is weak or non-existent orgasms. Men experience less stamina and weaker ejaculations. The weakening of the pelvic floor muscles in women results in reduced sexual arousal and infrequent orgasms. The lesson here is that if you want a better sex life, pay attention to your posture.

When you become more conscious of your posture, your body awareness will be sharper. You will notice areas of tightness and imbalance as you work to improve your posture. This sensitivity to trouble spots will help you get the most from my program. You will be able to choose the stretches you need to reduce pain and to build strength where you need it.

A REMINDER OF THE WAY TO STAND

I gave you general posture guidelines in chapter 2. Remember ears aligned with the shoulders and shoulder blades retracted or pulled closer together? The visualization of a string attached to the top of your head pulling you up gave you a simple way to improve how you stand. Because posture is so important to the health of your spine, I am giving you a more specific way to check your posture.

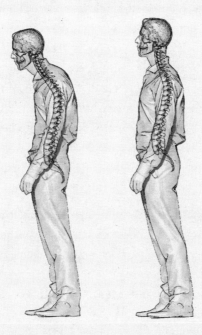

The following list breaks down proper posture body part by body part:

- Stand up straight and tall, your earlobes in line with your shoulders.

- Pull shoulders down and back.

- Keep your head level. Do not tilt your head forward, backward, or to the side.

- Let your arms hang naturally down the sides of your body.

- Tuck in your stomach.

- Keep your feet shoulder width apart.

- Balance your weight evenly on both feet.

- Keep your knees slightly bent.

- If you have to stand for a long time, shift your weight from the balls of your feet to your heels, or one foot to the other.

Be sure not to overcorrect by pulling your shoulders back too far. Trying to stand ramrod straight like a soldier creates muscle tension, stiffness, and pain in the upper back. By lifting your chest military-style, you overextend your lower back, which makes those lower back muscles work too hard.

Improving your posture begins with being mindful of how you are standing during the day. Stop regularly to notice how you are holding yourself. If you are slouching or jutting your head forward, realign your posture. Do not stay in one position for a long period of time. To prevent muscle fatigue, shift your position or get up to move every half hour to an hour.

ON SITTING

When you think about it, you probably spend a good deal of time sitting. If you are hunched over, you reverse some of your spine's natural curves. To realign your spine, sit upright as far back in your chair as you can with your feet flat on the floor. Your chin should be parallel to the floor and your shoulders relaxed. Be aware of the curve in your lower back. Do not allow that curve to flatten. Use a lumbar pillow or a rolled towel to maintain the lumbar curve.

A SIMPLE WAY TO FIND GOOD SITTING POSTURE

This quick exercise will help you to get into the right sitting position for spinal alignment:

- Sit slouching at the edge of your chair.

- Remember that string on the top of your head? Draw yourself up and accentuate the lower curve of your back as far as you can. Hold that position for a few seconds.

- Release the position about 10 degrees. This is how your spine should feel when you sit.

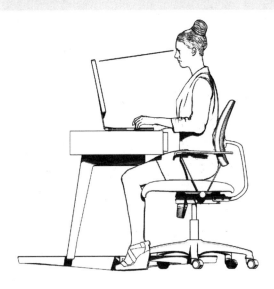

The Way to Sit

- Distribute your weight evenly on both hips.

- Your knees should be bent at a right angle. Your feet should be flat on the floor, and your knees even or slightly higher than your hips. Do not cross your legs.

- Relax your shoulders.

- Keep your elbows close to your body. Your elbows should be bent between 90 and 120 degrees.

- Your thighs should be parallel to the floor.

- Make sure your back is fully supported. Use a back pillow if your chair does not have a backrest to support your back's lower curve.

- Avoid sitting in the same position for more than thirty minutes.

- At work, adjust your chair height so that you can sit comfortably in this position.

- You should be able to be close to your work and tilt your computer up at you. Looking up can cause as much neck pain as looking down.

- Rest your elbows and arms on your chair or desk while keeping your shoulders relaxed.

- If your chair rolls and pivots, don't twist at the waist while sitting. Turn your whole body instead.

- When getting up, move to the front of the chair. With an erect back, straighten your legs to stand up. Do not bend forward at the waist.

SHOULDERS BACK

Irene, a seventy-year-old woman, came to see me with a particular postural problem. She was five feet, two inches tall, with a petite frame, and could not turn her head to see correctly when she was driving. Irene found it increasingly difficult to see the highway to drive safely. She was also upset because she was developing a hump just below her neck. Noticing her forward head posture, I realized poor posture was the root of her problem. I explained that proper posture involves a neutral spine, ears aligned with the shoulders, and angel wings, or shoulder blades, pulled toward each other to open the chest. In contrast, the ears are in front of the shoulders with poor posture, and the shoulders droop forward.

I recommended physical therapy for postural correction. The physical therapist trained her for an improved range of motion. The goal of range-of-motion training was to teach her how to use her spine joints again and then bring her head back. Irene performed stretches and Chest Openers. Her regimen progressed to using pulleys for strengthening her chest muscles. In time, the combination of awareness and building up her strength enabled her to correct her head-jutting-forward posture. Her spinal alignment improved significantly.

Irene learned a trick to correct her posture from her physical therapist. If she tucked her chin, which corrected her head jutting forward, then her rotational motion naturally improved. This way, Irene was better able to drive and observe the rotational visibility of the highway by looking over her shoulders and checking her blind spots. She found that if she used a lumbar support pillow, scooted her buttocks forward, and raised her car seat, her improved sitting posture allowed her to have a better view of the road while driving. Irene was happy with her newfound ease of driving, ability to look over each shoulder, and improved visibility of the road in front of her.

CHAIR CHOICES

If you spend your working hours sitting at a desk, using an ergonomic chair could help to reduce back problems. The ideal office chair has a lumbar adjustment for height and depth to provide a proper fit for supporting the inward curve of your lower back. An adjustable seat height is important so that your feet are flat on the floor. Another desirable feature is an adjustable forward or backward tilt in the seat of the chair.

Alternatives to traditional office chairs have become popular. They are designed to promote good posture and support your spine. These chairs can help you if you experience lower back pain. The nontraditional chairs include the:

Kneeling Ergonomic Chair

This office chair looks like a contraption. It has no back and you use it by sitting in a modified kneeling position. The design slides the hips forward, aligning the back, shoulders, and neck. It encourages good posture. The main support is from the seat of the chair and from the shins. Weight is distributed between the pelvis and the knees, which reduces spinal compression. Stress and tension in the lower back and leg muscles are also reduced. The chair has a forward slanting seat that creates a more natural position for the spine. Though it might take some time to get used to it, this type of office chair makes sitting in the proper position automatic and comfortable.

Exercise Ball Chair

Using an exercise ball as a desk or computer chair is another ergonomic option. The ball has to be large enough to support you. The balls come in various sizes, so you can find one that is the proper height for you. The chair encourages movement and active sitting. A slight bounce keeps your legs moving, which stimulates circulation and fires up your muscles. This reduces fatigue and stress. If you are sitting on a ball, slouching is near impossible. Staying on the ball automatically improves posture. Some of these chairs have a base frame with wheels for mobility and/or a backrest.

AT-HOME CHAIRS FOR BACK PAIN

Stay away from chairs without back support, stools for example, which make it difficult to remain sitting erect. The same is true for egg chairs. Hard, straight-backed chairs are also taboo if you have back problems because the straight back does not support the back's lumbar curve. Lumbar support is especially important. If there is a gap between your lower back and the chair, use a pillow for support. Armrests help to take the strain from your upper spine and shoulders. A footrest helps to reduce stress on the hips and spine.

Recliner

Studies have shown that rather than leaning forward or sitting upright, reclining at a 135-degree angle produces less disc movement in the spine, which can help with back pain. A recliner supports the entire back. Sitting in a reclined position is especially helpful for those with pain from lumbar spinal stenosis or degenerative disc disease.

Of course, a recliner is great for watching TV, but some use a recliner while working. Small tables are available that attach to the chair and can be pulled over the chair to allow for working on a laptop or paperwork.

Lift Chairs

A lift chair uses electric power to tilt and lift the entire chair. This makes it easier to get out of the chair and move around.

Zero-Gravity Chair

In this type of chair, your feet are at the same level as your heart when you recline. The position minimizes the toll that gravity takes on your body. A zero-gravity chair reduces strain on your vertebrae and decompresses your spine, relieves back pain, improves circulation, and cushions sore muscles. Like an astronaut, you will feel weightless and experience deep relaxation as well.

Massage and Heat Chair

What could be better than having a massage therapist available in your home 24/7? A common cause of back pain is tight, overworked muscles. A massage chair works to relax your muscles by stimulating the blood flow to areas of your back that need more oxygen and nutrients. This is especially helpful if you experience muscle spasms. Many massage chairs use heat as well. Warming up the area where muscles are tight can relax them.

When your muscles are strained, the stress on your skeleton is increased. Many massage chairs stretch and knead the problem areas where your muscles are too tight. Relaxing those muscles will help to reduce the stress on your skeletal structure, including your spine. Relaxing those muscles will help with spine alignment.

POSTURE CORRECTING STRETCHES

Your heightened posture awareness will produce change if you address the flaws in your posture with exercises and stretches to correct them. There is only so much simply paying attention to your posture will do. Years of bad posture probably have created imbalances in your body. To correct posture faults and realign your spine, you need to stretch shortened muscles and strengthen muscles, ligaments, and tendons that can become elongated and weakened by the stress bad posture puts on your spine.

An important component of the Watch Your Back program is the Posture Correcting Stretches, which everyone should do with the aging spine in mind. The workout consists of seven simple stretches and exercises to realign and strengthen your entire spine. The workout takes less than ten minutes if you do all the exercises. You might want to choose exercises targeted to a specific problem area, but it is best to begin by doing the full workout. These exercises will make a significant contribution to slowing the degeneration of your spine.

Half-Kneeling Hip Flexor Stretch

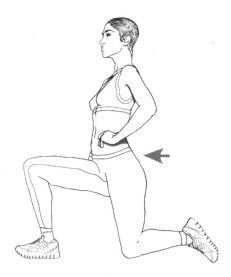

Hip flexors, a group of four muscles, are located on the front top part of your thigh in the pelvic area. They keep the posterior pelvic muscles in balance, which helps you to maintain good posture and prevents your pelvis from tilting forward. Hip flexors are activated every time you take a step. Sitting at a desk all day shortens and tightens these muscles, which results in the stiffness and soreness of "tight hips." Shortened muscles do not generate as much power as lengthened muscles. Weakened hip flexors strain and tear more easily. Strong flexors alleviate lower back pain and improve posture. This stretch will help to reverse the effects of sitting too long by lengthening the hip flexors.

- Kneel down and step your left foot forward in a lunge with both knees bent at 90 degrees. Contract your glutes so that your pelvis tilts beneath you slightly.

- Push your hips forward until you feel a stretch in the front of your right hip and down your thigh. Make sure your spine is tall. Avoid arching your back. Your hips should be in line with the length of your spine.

- Relax into the stretch. Hold 30 to 60 seconds as you breathe slowly. Relax and repeat 3 times.

- Repeat the stretch with your right foot forward. Hold for 30 to 60 seconds. Relax and repeat 3 times.

Wall Angels

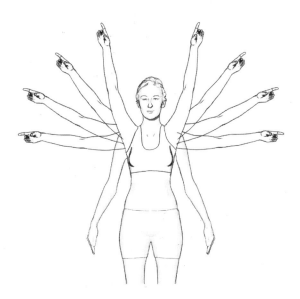

This stretch is like making snow angels in the winter. It is a deep, dynamic stretch for the spine. The movement strengthens back muscles and lengthens muscles in the front of the neck, shoulders, and core. By focusing on upper body mobility, Wall Angels promote proper spine alignment, strengthen muscles that hold the shoulders back, and help maintain a full range of motion. Wall Angels can reduce rounded shoulders by stretching the muscles in the front of the body. By working the upper and mid-spine, the vertebral joints in the neck may decompress, which relieves pain and tension and reduces jutting head.

- Stand with your back to the wall. Walk your feet out so that your heels are 6 inches from the wall.

- Lean back against the wall. Tuck your pelvis so that your lower back is against the wall. Pull your shoulders and head back to touch the wall.

- Slowly raise your arms overhead with their backs skimming the wall, until your hands touch overhead.

- Slowly lower your arms to the starting position. Make sure the backs of your arms never leave the wall.

- Repeat 5 to 10 times.

Chest Opener

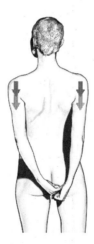

If you spend most of the day sitting slouched, your chest moves inward because your chest muscles are shortened and weakened. Your shoulders roll forward and your upper back rounds. Opening up your chest counteracts a rounded back. This stretch strengthens back and shoulder muscles for posture. With a reduction of tension, soreness and tightness are alleviated. No more slouching is where you want to end up.

- Stand with your feet hip-width apart.

- Bring your arms behind you and interlace your fingers with your palms pressing together. If your hands don't reach each other grasp a towel or exercise band.

- Keep your head, neck, and spine aligned as you look straight ahead.
- Inhale as you lift your chest toward the ceiling and bring your hands toward the floor.
- Breathe deeply as you hold the pose for 5 breaths.
- Release and relax for a few breaths.
- Repeat 5 to 10 times.

Isometric Rows

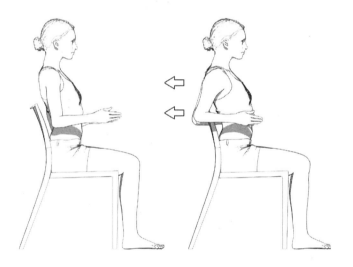

You can do this exercise sitting or standing. Isometric exercise involves contracting muscles without movement in surrounding joints. Holding one position stabilizes muscles, which stay at a constant length.

The rows strengthen shoulder, arm, and back muscles as well as tendons and ligaments. Isometric Rows relieve pain and stiffness.

- Sitting in a chair or standing, bend your arms with your fingers pointed forward and your palms facing each other.
- Exhale as your draw your elbows back and squeeze your shoulder blades together.

- Hold this position for 10 seconds breathing deeply.

- On an inhale, slowly release to starting position.

- Repeat this row 10 times.

Side Bends

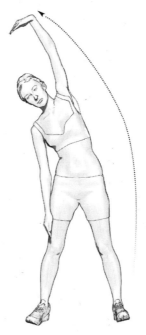

Side Bends improve posture and flexibility. If you spend a lot of time sitting crouched at a desk, your lateral back muscles shorten and feel tighter. The postural imbalance builds up stress in the lateral back, muscles, and hips. This imbalance results in more than back pain. It can restrict your lungs and affect your breathing.

The side-to-side motion, or lateral flexion, improves the flexibility of the lower back and abdominals, resulting in better support for the spine and improved posture. Side Bends improve core body strength, which is a key to good posture.

- Stand with your spine erect, your feet slightly apart, and your arms relaxed by your sides.

- Keeping your palms facing down, lift your right arm straight up to your shoulder.

- Turn your palm to face upward and reach your right arm vertically overhead.

- As you exhale, bend your upper body to the left and slide your left arm down your left leg as you do so.

- Hold the stretch for 30 seconds.

- On an inhale, return to the starting position and repeat the process on the other side.

- Repeat 10 times.

Glute Squeeze

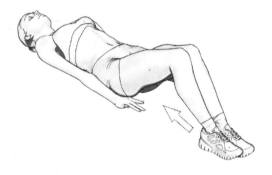

The gluteal muscles, popularly known as glutes, consist of the three muscles that make up the buttocks: the gluteus maximus, gluteus medius, and gluteus minimus. The muscles are responsible for extension, abduction (moves outward), and internal rotation of the legs and the hip joints. The glutes keep the hips healthy. Sitting too long creates an imbalance between the hip flexors and glutes. The flexors tighten and shorten, and the glutes lengthen and do not fire. When the glutes are weak, the muscles in the lower back and hamstrings take up the slack, which produces strain and pain. This isometric exercise strengthens and activates the glutes. With increased power, endurance, and strength, the glutes improve the alignment of the hips and pelvis, which means better posture and fewer aches and pains.

- Lie on your back with your knees bent and your feet about hip distance apart.

- Keep your feet about 12 inches from your hips. Your arms should be alongside your body with your palms facing down.

- As you exhale, tighten your glutes and bring your feet closer to your hips.

- Hold this position for 10 seconds, and then relax and return your feet to starting position.

- Repeat this movement for 1 minute.

Happy Baby Pose

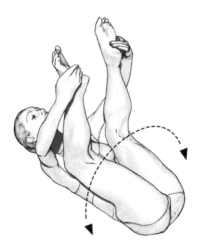

Aside from being fun to do, the Happy Baby Pose has many benefits. A hip opener, the stretch makes the hips more flexible and the pelvis stronger to support the spine. By strengthening the lower back muscles, this yoga pose relieves lower back pain. The pose realigns and stretches the spine, hips, glutes, hamstrings, and shoulder muscles. It relieves back and neck pain as well.

The stretch has a wonderful psychological component. Gentle and calming, the Happy Baby Pose increases relaxation and eases stress, anxiety, and fatigue. This is an all-around great stretch.

- Lie on your back, your head flat on the floor.

- Bend your knees toward your chest at a 90-degree angle with the soles of your feet facing upward to the ceiling.

- Reach forward and hold the insides or outsides of your feet. Do not lift your shoulders. If you cannot keep your shoulders flat, hold your ankles or shins instead of your feet.

- Spread your knees apart and shift them toward your armpits.

- Flex your heels into your hands and gently rock from side-to-side. Do this for up to 1 minute.

THE 4 POSTURE PROBLEMS

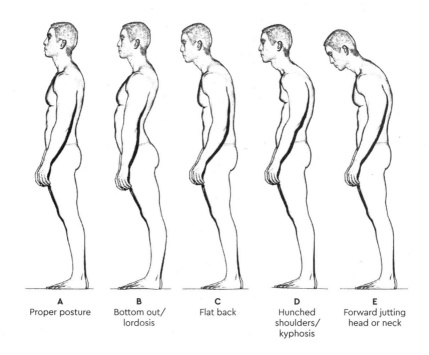

A	B	C	D	E
Proper posture	Bottom out/ lordosis	Flat back	Hunched shoulders/ kyphosis	Forward jutting head or neck

The illustration above shows the most common types of bad posture: bottom out/lordosis, flat back, hunched shoulders/kyphosis, and forward jutting head or neck.

A healthy, properly aligned spine is shaped like an S. The curves work like a coiled spring to maintain balance, absorb shock, and allow movement. Your abdominal muscles along with your back muscles help to maintain the S shape. As you can see graphically from the illustration above, poor posture changes the S shape, which has serious consequences for your spine and overall health.

After a discussion of each posture type, you will find a list of posture fixes, exercises, and stretches from elsewhere in the book that are particularly helpful for that condition. The page on which the stretch or exercise appears is indicated.

Bottom Out (Lordosis)

With bottom out posture, the curve in your lower spine is exaggerated, curving too far inward. You can see why this posture goes by the nickname "Donald Duck" posture. People who stand this way appear to be sticking out their stomach and butt. The curve of the neck shifts inward, which causes the head to tilt forward and the shoulders farther back. The condition can be caused by obesity, pregnancy, osteoporosis, wearing high heels, and sleeping on your stomach. Bottom out posture weakens core/stomach muscles.

To correct a sticking-out bottom, focus on core and buttock strengthening exercises and hip flexor and thigh stretches.

Fixes:

- Half-Kneeling Hip Flexor Stretch (see page 86)
- Plank (see page 175)
- Lying Lateral Leg Lifts (see page 174)
- Child's Pose (see page 179)

Flat Back

With this posture, the spine becomes flat and loses its natural lower curve, often due to muscle imbalances. Back or leg pain can result. A flat back makes you lean your neck and head forward, which can cause neck and upper back strain.

Any condition that shortens the front part of the spine, such as degenerative disc disease, herniated disc disease, and compression fractures, can cause the flat back posture. Prolonged sitting or bending can result in pain or discomfort for those with a flat back.

To correct a flat back, I recommend exercises to strengthen your core, buttocks, neck, and rear shoulder muscles.

Fixes:

- Plank (see page 175)
- Lying Lateral Leg Lifts (see page 174)
- Corner Stretch (see page 173)
- Chest Opener (see page 88)
- Cat-Cow Stretch (see page 169)

Hunched Shoulders (Kyphosis)

This condition results in forward rounding of the upper back region. With kyphosis, people stand with their shoulders forward, head down, and upper back curved. It puts a lot of pressure on the back and neck, resulting in neck pain and stiff upper back and shoulders. Kyphosis is common in older women who have osteoporosis as well as those who spend too much time hunched in front of computer screens, which should be at eye level, so you do not have to look down. Remember text neck.

Fixes:

- Plank (see page 175)
- Bridge (see page 170)
- Corner Stretch (see page 173)
- Chest Opener (see page 88)
- Cobra (see page 172)

HABITS THAT HURT

Text Neck

This chapter opened with my text neck study for a reason. Judging from the global response when the study was made public, I have to assume that many people are experiencing the consequences of time spent looking down at phones, tablets, handheld gaming systems, and other devices. The cell phone launched in 1983. I find it astonishing that our electronic culture created this widespread posture problem in less than forty years.

Looking down promotes forward head posture. The extra stress puts pressure on the front of the neck and gaps in the spine. This can cause the discs between the vertebrae to move backward, which increases the chances of disc bulges. The back of the neck is strained because the muscles on the backside are in a constant state of contraction in the attempt to support the head and pull it back. The upper back muscles become elongated and the chest muscles shorten. Text neck creates tightening in the front of the neck and chest, which affects the shoulders and middle back.

I know you are not about to give up your cell phone because of a pain in your neck. Making a few adjustments in the way you use your phone will help. One obvious change is to raise the phone and other devices closer to eye level to avoid tilting your head. Another is to take frequent breaks when you use handheld devices. During the breaks, you can arch your neck and upper back backward to counter your head-forward posture.

Regular exercise is important. A flexible, strong back and neck are better able to handle the extra stress caused by text neck. The following exercises will help to alleviate the pain and stiffness.

Fixes:

- Neck Tilts (see page 136)
- Neck Rotations (see page 136)
- Wall Angels (see page 87)
- Chest Opener (see page 88)
- Cobra (see page 172)

Slouching in Chair

If you slouch in a chair for hours every day, your spine will suffer the same effects as slouching while standing, but there are other potential problems that you might not expect. Slouching while sitting can lead to stress incontinence when you cough or laugh. When you slouch, there is more pressure on your stomach, which in turn puts pressure on the bladder. Slouching in a chair makes it more difficult for the muscles of the pelvic floor to hold against the additional pressure. Slouched sitting posture after a meal can slow digestion and cause heartburn and acid reflux.

You cannot forget about your posture while sitting. Maintaining a neutral, upright spine position for the hours you spend sitting each day is essential for good health.

Fixes:

- Chest Opener (see page 88)
- Bridge (see page 170)
- Cat-Cow Stretch (see page 169)
- Plank (see page 175)
- Cobra (see page 172)

Cradling a Phone with Shoulder

Do you hold your phone between your ear and shoulder at work to keep your hands free to type on the keyboard, or at home when you answer the phone while sautéing onions or holding the baby? Your body was not designed to hold the position for very long. If cradling your phone is a habit, you are straining the muscles of your neck, upper back, and shoulders. Holding such an unnatural position can lead to muscle imbalances between the left and right side of your neck.

Fixes:

- Wall Angels (see page 87)
- Chest Opener (see page 88)
- Isometric Rows (see page 89)
- Head Drop and Raise (see page 135)
- Neck Rotations (see page 136)

Improving your posture is the first strategy of the program because the way you stand and sit has such a powerful impact on your spine and overall health. Good posture provides the foundation on which you build a strong and flexible back. The Posture Correcting Stretches and posture fixes in this chapter will get you on track. The exercises and stretches are part of the daily program. As you begin your efforts to improve your posture, remember that changing your posture can be the most effective painkiller you can find.

Chapter 5

Strategy 2:
Take a Deep Breath

There is a reason you take a deep breath before you are about to do something challenging. That slow, full breath calms you down and centers you. Conscious, deep breathing can relieve all kinds of tension and has many more benefits for your mind and body.

Remember the "fight-or-flight" response? When you are under a lot of stress, you are likely to take short, shallow breaths. Your heart rate and blood pressure rise, and your muscles tighten. Not enough oxygenated air reaches the lowest part of your lungs, which can make you feel anxious. When you take deep, belly-expanding breaths, your physical and emotional responses to stress change.

Deep breathing encourages a full oxygen exchange. When you inhale, oxygen moves from the lungs to the bloodstream. At the same time carbon dioxide passes from the blood to the lungs. When you breathe deeply, this exchange of gases has more volume. This fuller trade can slow your heartbeat, lower your blood pressure, and reduce muscle tension. In short, slowing your breathing relaxes your body, which has a positive effect on your spine.

Controlled, slow breathing is also called belly breathing, diaphragmatic breathing, or abdominal breathing. When you breathe deeply, you engage your diaphragm, which is a domed shaped muscle located at the bottom of your ribcage. When you inhale, your diaphragm tightens and moves downward. This action creates more space in your chest cavity into which the lungs can expand to take in more air. Creating even more room for your lungs to inflate, muscles between your ribs raise your rib cage.

When you exhale, your diaphragm relaxes and moves upward in your chest, pushing out the carbon dioxide. A deeper inhalation allows more oxygen to create energy throughout your body.

WHAT BELLY BREATHING CAN DO FOR YOU

Stopping to be aware of the rhythm and rate of your breath is a proven way to ease your back pain. Instead of focusing on the pain, you concentrate on your breath. Your pain takes a back seat when it is not the center of your attention. Directing attention away from your suffering distances you from the pain. If you focus on your breath, your experience of pain decreases. I have to add that the physical movement of deep breathing is an instant posture fix.

Diaphragmatic breathing has many direct, physical benefits as well. You might think I am over-promising, but the benefits, which follow, are scientific fact.

Releases Endorphins

During deep abdominal breathing, the increased oxygen in your blood triggers the release of endorphins and enkephalins, which are associated with more than happy, positive feelings. These hormones are the body's natural painkillers. They send "stop pain" messages in your body. That is great news if you are suffering from chronic back pain.

Reduces Anxiety and Stress

Deep breathing is a very effective relaxation technique. The increase of the supply of oxygen to your brain stimulates the parasympathetic nervous system, which is responsible for the body's "rest-and-digest" response. The parasympathetic nervous system undoes the work of the sympathetic system's "fight-or-flight" response to a stressful situation. The parasympathetic nervous system reduces stress hormones in your blood, decreases the elevated respiration and heart rate of the stress response, and decreases muscle tension. By quieting the stress response, belly breathing helps to reduce inflammation in the body. This takes your body from a state of high alert to calmness, from stress and anxiety to a feeling of well-being. Since stress is a major trigger of back problems, quieting your body's stress response will help alleviate your back pain.

Increases Lymphatic Flow

The lymphatic system is an important part of your immune system. It is responsible for protecting your body from illness-causing invaders, maintaining body fluid levels, and removing cellular waste. Unlike the blood circulatory system, the lymphatic system does not have an active pump like the heart to propel lymphatic fluid into the bloodstream. The system relies on muscle activity. The up and down movement of the diaphragm during deep abdominal breathing helps to return lymphatic fluid to the bloodstream. Stimulating the lymphatic system increases the rate at which waste products are removed from the body through the lymphatic flow. Removing waste products more efficiently from the body reduces swelling and increases muscle strength, both of which promote healing.

Warms Up Your Spine

In addition to shifting your focus from pain to your breathing, this relaxation technique contributes to spinal health. To begin with, every deep breath you take naturally mobilizes the spine. If you take a deep breath in, allow the diaphragm to descend and the chest wall to expand, the thoracic spine moves into extension. As you exhale deeply and relax, the thoracic spine flexes. Deep breathing is a warm-up for the spine.

Improves Spine's Mobility and Reduces Inflammation in Spinal Nerves

As you have learned, abdominal breathing decreases inflammation and swelling, which improves the motion of your spinal joints, cord, and nerve roots. When spinal nerves are able to move in the nerve canal with each breath, inflamed nerves heal themselves. Pain goes away, or is at least reduced, when nerves are no longer inflamed.

Hydrates Discs

Back pain and spine problems are unexpected results of dehydration. The spine, especially the discs, holds a surprising amount of water. When your discs are dehydrated, they lose volume, which increases the chances of degeneration and injury. Deep breathing sends more blood to the spine, improving disc hydration, which enables healing oxygen and nutrition to travel to the discs and joints.

Improves the Health of the Central Nervous System

Cerebrospinal fluid (CSF), a clear, colorless liquid, fills and surrounds the brain and the spinal cord. The liquid provides a life jacket for the brain and spinal cord, a barrier against shock. Though the primary function of CSF is to cushion the brain within the skull and serve as a shock absorber for the central nervous system, the CSF regulates the chemical environment of the brain. CSF circulates nutrients and chemicals filtered from the blood and removes waste products from the brain. The fluid also transports metabolic waste products, antibodies, chemicals, and pathological products of disease away from the brain and spinal cord into the bloodstream. Because the brain does not have a lymphatic system, the movement of the lungs, as well as the pulse of the heart, generate the movement of the CSF. When you breathe deeply, the motion and distribution of CSF increases, and that is a good thing.

Now you know why belly breathing is one of the strategies of my program. Nothing could be more basic than breathing. You have been doing it without interruption since the first breath you took. If you are like most people, breathing does not get a lot of your attention. The fact is that if you bring your attention to your breathing and learn to control it for just a few minutes a day, you will have a powerful tool against stress and back pain.

THE MAGIC OF DEEP BREATHING

Caitlyn is a forty-one-year-old professor of fine arts who suffered back pain and left-sided sciatica for years. I observed during her first visit that she was perspiring, restless, and irritable, all symptoms of anxiety. Her MRI and X-rays showed mild to moderate spinal stenosis at L4-L5. We set about introducing Caitlyn to the strategies of the Watch Your Back program.

On a subsequent visit, I was delighted to learn that Caitlyn's back pain had been significantly reduced. Amazed by the improvements, Caitlyn wanted to know how simply doing deep belly breathing for about ten minutes a day had relieved her back pain and anxiety.

I reminded Caitlyn that she was doing a lot more to calm her spine and mind. She had become more conscious of how she was moving. Caitlyn was making an effort to avoid bending, lifting, twisting and reaching, movements that could inflame her spine and nerves.

She insisted that the breathing was a magical pain reliever. I explained that when you breathe deeply, with belly motions in and out, the diaphragm pushes and pulls the lungs to the total capacity. The deep breaths you take lead to better oxygenation of the body, which diminishes anxiety and makes you feel good. When you are sad or in pain, you tend to take shallow breaths. As a result, you are only partially oxygenated.

At the same time, breathing profoundly moves you into proper posture, which helps to reduce pain. Deep belly breaths move and massage the spinal fluid around your spinal cord and the spine's nerve roots. The spinal nerves communicate with the brain and relay messages to the rest of your body.

"Who would have thought that breathing could do so much," Caitlyn responded with enthusiasm. "I will make deep breathing a lifelong habit." She grinned and asked, "What other tricks do you have up your sleeve, Dr. Ken?"

THREE DEEP BREATHING TECHNIQUES FOR BACK PAIN

What is especially appealing about deep breathing is that this calming technique is available to you anytime, anyplace. You can even practice deep breathing without others being aware that you are doing it.

To give you options, I will describe three different techniques: classic diaphragmatic breathing, my Count to Five deep breathing technique, and back-opening breathing.

Warning: If you are new to controlled, deliberate breathing, you may feel dizzy or lightheaded after a few breaths. As you become more experienced, you will be able to practice longer without dizziness.

If you do feel lightheaded, sit or lie still for a minute and resume normal breathing.

Belly Breathing

I have observed that many of my patients habitually breathe only with their chests. Poor posture and stress contribute to shallow breathing. Learning to breathe from the belly helped them to manage their back pain.

- You can practice belly breathing sitting in a chair or lying on your back. Find a quiet, comfortable place.

- If you are sitting in a chair, your head, neck, and shoulders should be relaxed. Though your posture does not have to be rigid, you want to avoid slouching, which will interfere with taking a deep breath.

- If you are lying down, you can bend your knees if it is more comfortable. You can use a small pillow under your head and knees as well.

- Place one hand on your upper chest and the other below your ribcage, right above your navel. As you breathe in and out, the hand on your upper chest should not move much. The hand on your belly should move with the breathing motion of your diaphragm.

- Inhale through your nose. Breathe in slowly and smoothly. As you feel the air move downward, your stomach should rise with your hand, while the hand on your chest barely moves at all. Avoid forcing or pushing your abdominal muscles outward.

- Breathe out slowly through your mouth with pursed lips. Try to exhale at least twice as long as you inhale. Let your belly relax. The hand on your stomach should move inward toward your spine. Again, the hand on your chest should be comparatively still.

When you are beginning to do belly breathing, try to repeat the breath sequence three times. Start slowly and build up gradually. You can work up to repeating belly breathing for five to ten minutes, one or two times a day.

COUNT TO FIVE

Nicole is a thirty-six-year-old mother of four children. She had profound anxiety attacks and a panic disorder. This patient suffered neck and shoulder pain and needed help. She was anxious to be evaluated. Her persistent pain was interfering with the attention she was able to give to her children. Her husband had pitched in, but she felt awful and guilty. She wanted to be there for her children. She told me she had anxiety and panic attacks. She was accustomed to living with it. As we talked, she began hyperventilating. I could see that stress had overwhelmed her.

I came from behind my desk and sat down in a chair next to her. I asked her to trust me to help her calm her anxiety. I demonstrated my Count to Five deep belly breathing technique, which has helped many of my patients. I told her to:

Breathe deeply in through your nose.

Feel your belly rise in five incremental steps.

Breathe deeply for a count of five. As you breathe in, feel your belly rise.

1 . . . 2 . . . 3 . . . 4 . . . 5 . . .

Hold your breath for a few seconds.

Exhale through your mouth.

Feel your belly fall in five incremental steps.

1 . . . 2 . . . 3 . . . 4 . . . 5 . . .

I did this routine with her for five minutes. When we stopped, my patient was visibly calmer. Nicole sighed with relief and thanked me. She became a convert to the power of deep breathing. We were able to proceed with our first consultation. I took her story, examined her, and sent her for the relevant tests. Now Nicole has an effective tool to help her deal with her next panic attack.

Back-Opening Exercise

This belly breathing technique will improve your posture as well as reduce your back pain. You can do this exercise in any position—standing, sitting, kneeling, lying down on your back, side-lying, or lying on your belly—as long as you are comfortable, and your weight is evenly distributed. Sitting in a relaxed, upright position is a good way to start.

As you do this breathing exercise, you should begin to feel a difference in the length of your spine, the release of neck and shoulder tension, and the support of your low abdominal muscles.

- Breathe in deeply through your nose and think of the air moving down toward your tailbone.

- Continue to inhale until you feel the air traveling up the ribcage, lifting the ribs off the hips.

- As you breathe out, pull your lower abs up and back toward your bottom back ribs.

- When you finish breathing out, allow your shoulder blades to drop down, which will lengthen your upper back and float your neck and head up.

Begin by doing this breathing sequence four times. Gradually build up to doing this breath for five to ten minutes a day.

You might want to try all three breathing techniques to see which one works best for you. My patients have had great results from practicing my Count to Five technique. As you deep breathe, avoid trying too hard, which may make you tense up. Your breath has to be your focal point. Deep breathing works because you shift your focus from what is stressing you to the deep, calm rhythms of your breath.

The beauty of belly breathing is that you can do it anywhere when you need to relax. You can practice deep breathing while you are doing other things. Try it while you are commuting, walking your dog, sitting at your desk at work, or in the waiting room of your doctor's office. It takes such a small amount of time to reap substantial benefits. A commitment to breathing deeply for less than two minutes a day can make a big difference in how you experience your back or neck pain.

Chapter 6

Strategy 3:
The Right Moves

Have you ever felt a ping in your back when you bend to pick something up, reach for a dish on a high shelf in the kitchen, or take heavy grocery bags from the trunk of your car? If you are not mindful about how you move, everyday activities—bending, lifting, lowering, turning, reaching overhead, pulling, and pushing—can injure your back or aggravate existing conditions. You have to move with your spine in mind. Moving the right way will help you to avoid back strains, sprains, and injuries. Poor body mechanics put you at high risk of developing back problems.

When you do not move correctly and safely, your spine is subjected to abnormal stresses that over time can lead to degeneration of discs and joints, injury, and unnecessary wear and tear. Many of my patients have jobs that require heavy lifting or repetitive motion. I treat people who drive for a living, construction workers, nurses and healthcare providers, office workers, manual laborers, dentists and dental hygienists, warehouse and distribution workers, auto mechanics, hairstylists, factory workers, teachers, and people involved in baby care. Their work takes a toll on their bodies. They come to see me experiencing varying degrees of pain. As part of their treatment, I make them aware of body mechanics, what they can do to reduce the stress that their movements on the job put on their spine. I have seen repeatedly that when my patients learn to move with proper body mechanics, they ease their back and neck pain, prevent flare-ups, and protect their back. This chapter will show you how to move with your spine in mind.

A LIFETIME OF LIFTING
1,000 POUNDS A DAY

Bill, at sixty-four, was almost ready to retire. He had worked for twenty-five years with an express delivery company. He complained about back pain and hamstring tenderness, which were getting worse.

We calculated his daily load of lifting. He carried an average of two hundred packages a day, weighing six ounces to fifty pounds. We estimated an average weight of 2.5 pounds per package. He loaded the boxes onto the truck and then delivered them. His daily lifting was two hundred packages x 2.5 pounds x twice a day. That comes to an estimated one thousand pounds of lifting each day. With the increased volume of holidays and online shopping, the number of packages he had to deliver every day was steadily rising.

I explained my concept of the 250 times magnifier. Whatever he lifted in a day, five days a week, fifty weeks a year, is a magnification of 250 times a day. If Bill lifts one thousand pounds a day, he is lifting 250,000 pounds a year. I have treated workers who routinely lift 6,000 pounds a day, which translates to 1.5 million pounds annually.

Carrying objects and packages close to your body will save your spine. Objects lifted by a delivery person exert multiplied forces on the spine. An object lifted close to the body may exert half the object's weight as a force to the spine. An object forty-five degrees away from the body exerts two times the force of the object's weight. Holding an object ninety degrees away from the body exerts four times the force of the object's weight.

My calculation made Bill realize he needed to warm up like an elite athlete for his workday. He practiced the Watch Your Back strategies of core strengthening for three months. Then Bill included deep breathing, stretching, strengthening, and aerobic warm-up before work. Bill was looking forward to retiring.

He was convinced that the Watch Your Back program would allow him to enjoy his retirement without pain, an achievement after a lifetime of lifting.

If you are over thirty, you have to pay particular attention to how you move. Of course, this is true no matter your age, but the risk of injuring your back becomes greater as the years pass. The older you are, the more likely you are to have a history of injured muscles, ligaments, or discs, which can make you vulnerable to further injury. In addition, your muscles and ligaments become less flexible and your discs more brittle with age. One false move could result in injury and long-lasting back pain.

This chapter demonstrates the right moves you need to make to avoid back pain. You will also learn how to protect your back when you cough or sneeze or face a long drive, which are often triggers for back pain.

BASIC GUIDELINES

There are three fundamental rules for protecting your spine when you move:

- Keep your backbone straight.
- Always have a wide base of support.
- Avoid bending and twisting your spine.

Proper Bending

If you bend at the waist or hips when you pick something up from the floor or take something from the trunk of your car, you could be asking for trouble. Your back looks like the letter C when you bend from the waist. Bending this way puts more stress on your spinal discs, which do not need additional wear and tear. Bad bending body mechanics transfer more forces and stresses to the lower back. This is the way to bend, which will save your back:

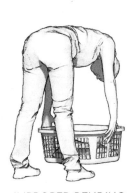
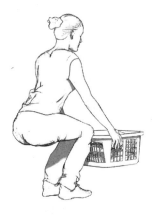

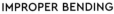
IMPROPER BENDING   PROPER BENDING

- Look straight ahead rather than looking down.

- Keep your head up and your spine straight.

- Pull in your stomach to engage your core.

- Bend your knees to lower your body slowly.

- Keep your feet about hip distance apart and your heels down and planted on the ground.

- Bring what you are picking up close to your center before you rise.

- Push up from your legs. Be sure to keep your back straight as you rise slowly.

- Keep the load at waist height, close to your body.

If you are getting something from the trunk of your car or a low table, similar rules apply:

- Do not bend from your waist. Squat by bending your knees.

- Maintain the natural curves of your back.

- Do not twist your body.

- If you have to lean forward, move your whole body, not just your arms, which would put considerable strain on your back.

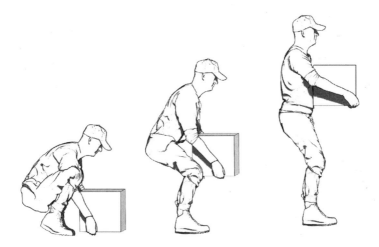

Proper Lifting

The rule to bend from the knees, not the waist, applies to lifting as well.

You should be realistic about your limits when you are about to lift something. If the object is too heavy, do not try to lift it alone. You will not get a gold medal for straining your back. Do not hesitate to get someone to help you.

Avoid twisting while you lift, which is a very risky move that could have painful consequences. If you need to turn, pivot your feet when you are upright.

It is a good idea to know where you plan to take what you are going to lift and how you will get it there. You do not want to run into obstructions while carrying something.

One back-saving rule: if you can, push instead of lift.

Finally, do not forget hand trucks, dollies, and carts. Using moving tools will save your back.

- Stand close to the object with your feet spread shoulder width apart for a strong base of support.

- Squat, bending your knees while keeping your back straight in proper alignment.

- Contract your stomach muscles to keep your back from over-arching.

- Take a deep breath and exhale as you lift.

- Lift with your legs by straightening them, not your back. Make sure not to lift or twist at the same time.

- Hold what you are lifting as close to your body as you can between your hips and your shoulders.

- Use smooth controlled movements as you lift.

- If you are lifting the object with someone else, do it in unison. One person should say when to lift, walk, and unload.

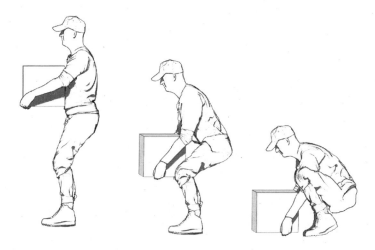

Proper Lowering

Lowering is the reverse of lifting. Just reverse the illustrations for proper lifting.

- Slowly bend your knees to lower the load.

- Keep your back straight and the weight close to the center of your body.

- If you are putting the load on a table, rest it on the edge and push it forward with your arms and body.

- If you are lowering the load to the floor, slowly bend your knees. Keep your back straight and the load close to your body as you squat.

Proper Turning

Have you noticed that moving from your waist is risky for your spine? Twisting affects the spinal facet joints in particular. Your vulnerable lower back ends up carrying the load when you twist from the waist.

- Pivot with your feet—don't twist at the waist.
- Maintain proper spine alignment.
- Allow for clearance.
- Keep the load in front of you.

Proper Reaching

It is common to look like a dancer when reaching for something. Do you stand on your toes? Raise one leg behind you? Stretch forward? That is not the way to go. An outstretched position causes traction of the nerve roots in the spinal canals. If you stand too far from what you are reaching for, the distance magnifies the forces on the spine. When you reach too far, your neck extends and your spinal canal narrows. If you stand closer, your spine is in flexion, which allows more space for the nerve roots.

When you are reaching for something, whether you are sitting or standing, the following rules apply:

- Position yourself close to the object you are trying to reach. Be as close as you can to avoid stretching. If you are standing, keep both of your feet on the ground.

- Avoid bending from the waist, twisting, or straining when reaching. If you are standing, position yourself by bending your knees.

- Let your arms and legs carry the weight, not your back.

THE HAZARDS OF REPETITION

When he was fifty-seven, Lawrence came to see me. He had worked as a house painter for thirty years, five years as a painter's apprentice and thirty years as a premiere painter, a true craftsman. Larry suffered from neck pain that radiated down his arms when he painted. Reaching was the worst thing he could do because it exacerbated his symptoms.

MRI and X-rays showed severe cervical stenosis at C4-C5, C5-C6, and C6-C7. Surgery was indicated to decompress the spinal cord and nerve roots. It was not easy to tell him that the severity of his problem, with three levels of fusion, made it necessary for him to consider retiring. I told him that if he continued to paint, he could wear out other cervical levels, a process called junctional stenosis. Larry knew he needed an operation but was not prepared to give up his profession. He focused on the fact that he needed to take care of his family and decided to delay surgery.

I began his treatment by introducing Larry to the Watch Your Back strategies. I told him that his primary concern was to avoid bending, lifting, twisting, and reaching, especially reaching, which he did for hours a day as he worked. Repetitive reaching aggravates cervical nerves, and worsens spinal cord compression, especially stenosis. I explained to him that repetitive reaching motions can cause nerves to be mobilized through tight canals, which leads to pain and discomfort. The act of reaching tends to make tight nerves symptomatic.

I explained that he had to correct his movement while he worked. If he positioned himself closer to his work with a ladder, instead of reaching up to paint, he would protect his nerves. Being closer to the job would keep him from extending his neck. Looking up created a tighter canal. If he leaned forward into a flexion position, he would create more space for his spinal cord and nerve roots. The shift in position would help to relieve his pain.

I advised him to take quick breaks regularly to do stretches while he was working or anytime the pain bothered him. For his problem, I suggested that he try Neck Tilts (see page 136), Neck Rotations (see page 136), Wall Angels (see page 87), Corner Stretch (see page 173), and Cobra (see page 172).

He needed to try some strengthening exercises to loosen up and strengthen his shoulders and core. I recommended doing Chest Openers (see page 88), Isometric Rows (see page 89), and Planks (see page 175).

I showed him the Count to Five deep belly breathing technique, which he practiced often during the day. He was able to do deep breathing as he painted. He told me that he could directly calm an irritated nerve with deep breaths. By moving higher on the ladder, he positioned his neck above the job, which eliminated extensive reaching. Larry was able to prolong his career another ten years.

When Larry finally retired, he agreed to have a cervical spine decompression and fusion operation, which I performed. Close to being pain free, he still uses the Watch Your Back strategies to maintain the comfort of his neck and arms. He is enjoying his retirement much more than he had expected to.

Proper Reaching Overhead

Reaching and taking something down from above your head can be a perilous undertaking. Taking these precautions will keep you from hurting yourself.

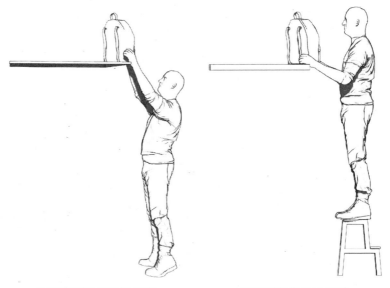

IMPROPER REACHING   PROPER REACHING

- Always check the weight of the load before moving it. Test by lifting one corner of what you want to get. When you plan to lift or lower an object from above your shoulders, lighten the load whenever possible.

- Position yourself close to the object you are trying to reach. Reach only as high as you can comfortably. Avoid stretching. Do not bend, twist, or strain when reaching.

- Put one leg in front of the other for support.

- Let your arms and legs carry the weight, not your back.

- Keep the load close to your body.

- Use a step stool if needed. Stand on something sturdy to get closer to what you want to reach above you.

- When you are lowering objects from above the shoulders, slide the load close to your body, grasp the object firmly, slide it down your body to your waist, and proceed with your move.

REPETITIVE MOTIONS

Proper Pulling and Pushing

Pushing is always a better bet than pulling. Pushing is a safer option for your back because it involves fewer muscles in the lower back. An added benefit: when you push you can see where you are going.

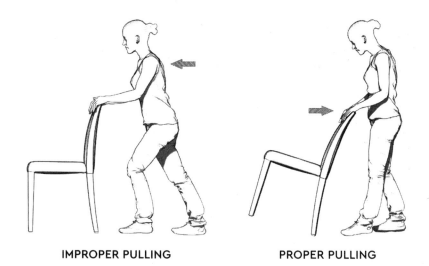

IMPROPER PULLING   PROPER PULLING

- Stay close to the load, do not lean forward. Never push or pull with a bent back.

- Push rather than pull whenever possible. You can push twice as much as you can pull without strain. When you push you tend to use your stomach muscles more than when you pull. Pulling puts more stress on your back.

- Use both arms.

- Tighten your stomach muscles when pushing.

- Do not twist. Keep your hips facing in the direction of the push.

- Always use your body weight and not your feet when pushing.

- If you are pulling, face the load. Facing forward and pulling an object behind you can lead to poor body mechanics, which increases your risk of injury. Facing the load allows you to use your body weight to pull an object safely.

Sudden Moves: Coughing, Sneezing, Yawning, and Laughing

Sometimes a coughing or sneezing fit, a big yawn, or even a good laugh can cause acute back pain or reignite a past problem. People tend to hunch their shoulders and lean forward when they do any of these seemingly harmless things. The movement of your body can put a strain on your back that leads to lower back pain or back spasms. A bad cough can stretch or tear a ligament. When your spine is flexed this way, the pressure on your discs increases significantly, which makes your discs vulnerable to injury. Compressed discs can tear, or existing tears can worsen. If you have a herniated disc, coughing can intensify the pain. Bending forward quickly and forcefully can create pressure on the spine's nerve roots, producing sudden acute back pain or can aggravate chronic pain.

There are two things you can do to protect yourself from cough-induced pain:

- Be mindful of your posture when you cough, sneeze, yawn, or laugh. Stop yourself from hunching forward. Make sure your spine keeps its natural shape to reduce pressure on your spinal discs.

- Support yourself. When you feel a cough coming, put your hands down on a firm, flat surface such as a table or ledge. This will stabilize you and decrease the compression of your spine.

Armed with this action plan, you can dodge a flare-up of back pain or an injury.

On the Road Again

Many of my patients complain about back pain on long road trips. If they find themselves sitting in traffic, even for short trips like going to work every day, driving seems to cause or intensify back pain for other patients. I decided to look into the effects of driving on the back.

In my research, I came across the phenomenon of whole-body vibration, which I will explain here in simple terms. When your car starts moving, your body experiences various forces, such as acceleration and deceleration and swaying from side to side. Whole body vibration occurs as your car travels over roads, and the vibrations transfer through the floor of the vehicle or seat into your legs and spine. Whole body vibration has been shown to cause musculoskeletal disorders, most commonly lower back pain. Aches and pains and weakness in the arm, shoulder, or the neck can develop as well.

Another aspect of driving that affects your back involves your feet. When your right foot is active on the accelerator pedal, your feet do not stabilize your lower body as they would while you sit in a chair with your feet on the floor. In the case of manual shifting, both feet are busy, and your stability can be compromised. As a result, your spine absorbs every bump, which is a formula for problems.

My patients tell me that the worst part of driving is the bumps in the road, which jar the spine. Before they hit the road, they do what they can to ensure a smooth ride. In preparation for a long trip, they make sure the car's shocks and tires are not worn. Some reduce tire pressure a bit. Others travel with driving accessories, such as a car seat cushion or a lumbar pillow. Some make sure to have a cold or heat pack with them just in case they need pain relief.

There are a number of things you can do to prevent back pain while driving:

- Keep your back pockets empty. Sitting on your wallet or phone may throw your spine out of alignment.

- Adjust your seat and headrest:

  ▸ Sit close to the steering wheel. For airbag safety, your chest should be at least ten inches from the steering wheel. If you sit too far from the steering wheel, reaching for it puts more stress on your lower back, neck, shoulders, and wrists.

▸ When you are close to the steering wheel, you will not have to strain to reach the pedals.

▸ If your knees are slightly higher than your hips, you will reduce the pressure on your lower back and hamstrings.

▸ Adjust the angle of your seatback to a 100- to 110-degree angle to sit properly. Your shoulders should be slightly behind your hips.

▸ The headrest should be in the middle of your head. To ensure good posture, your neck and back of your head should be in a neutral position.

▸ Add a lumbar support if necessary. If you do not have a support pillow, you can roll up a towel or a sweatshirt and place it in the small of your back for support.

• Adjust your mirrors so you don't have to twist to see them. You should only need to move your eyes to use the side mirrors. Always adjust them while you are sitting up straight. A changing view will alert you that you are slouching and need to correct your posture.

• Change your steering wheel grip. Because of airbags, experts suggest that your hands be at a nine o'clock and three o'clock position. This position allows you to rest your elbows on the armrests to prevent upper back pain.

• Use cruise control on long trips if you have it.

• If you have a heated seat, turn it on. The heat relaxes tight muscles. If your car does not have heated seats, you can buy a heated seat cover.

• Sitting in one position will stiffen up your back muscles. Achiness and muscle spasms can result. You should take a fifteen-minute break every two hours of driving. If you have back problems, you might want to take breaks more often, say every thirty minutes. You can pull over to the side of the road and safely get out of your car to move around and stretch, which will stimulate blood circulation to your lower back.

- Shift your position now and then. Between driving breaks, stretch and move in your seat. You can adjust your seat slightly every now and then. Any movement you can do safely will help to keep pain at bay.

- Save your back by getting in and out of the car the right way. Face away from the seat when you get in. Backside in, lower yourself carefully, sit, rotate to face front, and then slide in your feet. Be careful not to twist your back. To get out, scoot forward and swivel toward the door. Plant your feet on the ground, then raise yourself up. You can use the door frame for support if you need to.

Whether you bend and lift on the job, are on your feet teaching or nursing, or sit at your computer all day, moving the right way is the best defense against injuring your back. Knowing the biomechanics of good movement will protect you from sudden acute pain or chronic pain from long-term wear and tear. From how to move, the focus now shifts to breaking out of couch potato mode. The following chapter will convince you that you have to move more.

Chapter 7

Strategy 4:
Stand Up and Move

Think of how much time you spend sitting or lying down each day. How many of your waking hours do you sit at a desk, at a conference room table, in restaurants, in your car, on buses or trains? When you get home, do you lie on the sofa in front of the TV or sit at a computer screen? All the labor-saving devices in your life can contribute to your inactivity. You can shop with a click, change channels, open the garage door, and answer the phone without having to get up from your chair. There is not much required movement in a day.

American adults spend 55 to 70 percent of their time sitting or lying down, which would be 9.4 to 12 hours a day. If you add seven hours for sleep, you could be sedentary for as much as nineteen hours a day. So much inactivity is hazardous to your overall health and a disaster for your spine.

Sitting has become the new smoking. Research has shown that sitting or lying down for too long increases your risk of chronic health problems, such as heart disease, diabetes, and some cancers. Being sedentary can affect your mental health as well. If you stand or move during the day, you have a lower risk of early death than if you sit at a desk for hours without moving. If you have a sedentary lifestyle, you have a higher chance of being overweight, developing type 2 diabetes or heart disease, and experiencing depression and anxiety.

As for your spine, inactivity can increase swelling and contribute to malnourishment and degeneration in the discs. Discs do not have blood vessels. They depend on diffusion from blood vessels for nutrients, mainly glucose and oxygen, and the removal of metabolic waste, such as lactic acid. The fluid exchange helps to reduce the swelling in the other soft tissues surrounding injured discs. Exercise increases blood flow. The increased blood supply brings fresh oxygen to restore the discs and helps to wash away lactates and other byproducts of cellular metabolism.

TAKE AN ACTIVE BREAK
EVERY HOUR YOU SIT

The best way to avoid the negative effects of being sedentary is to make sure you stand up and move around for two to five minutes every hour. Standing takes pressure off your neck and lower back and increases circulation, especially to your lower extremities. An hourly active break is a perfect time to do a few posture-improving stretches (see page 134).

I could go on for pages about how bad inactivity is for you, but I would rather focus on the many benefits of increased physical activity. The most powerful way to combat stress is to move more. Exercise can refresh you by clearing your mind and emotions. Movement is a mood elevator. Improving the blood flow to your brain can put you in a mindset that promotes a more positive outlook on life. An active lifestyle will not only make you look and feel better, but your take on life will be more optimistic.

When you make exercise a part of your life, you will experience an overall sense of well-being. Your metabolism will pick up, and you can start to lose weight and keep it off. With a diminished reaction to stress, your sleep will improve. Exercise, which induces the release of "feel-good" chemicals from the brain, is known to alleviate depression and anxiety. Being active builds and maintains healthy bones, muscles, and joints. As you can see, exercise delivers benefits that fulfill the strategic goals of the Watch Your Back program.

Being physically active is good for the health of your spine. Exercise strengthens, stretches, and repairs muscles that help to support your back. Back and abdominal muscles buttress the vertebrae, discs, facet joints, and ligaments. When weak back and abdominal muscles cannot provide support, muscles, ligaments, and tendons become more vulnerable to strains and sprains. In addition, exercising the back reduces stiffness by keeping the connective fibers of ligaments and tendons flexible, which prevents tears, injury, and back pain.

One of the key strategies of my Watch Your Back program is to get up and start moving. Being a couch potato or chained to your desk is asking for trouble. I do not expect you to become a body builder or a marathon runner overnight to get healthy. You just have to be mindful of moving more in your day-to-day life. Increased movement will energize you, and that increased energy will motivate you to keep moving.

OFFICIAL GUIDELINES FOR PHYSICAL ACTIVITY

You escape the sedentary category if you do just thirty minutes of moderate exercise most days of the week, which means four days. In 2020, the U.S. Department of Health and Human Services published the recommended guidelines for physical activity, which give you a goal to aim for. You do not need to try to meet these goals on Day 1. The guidelines are the ideal. Nothing will be more likely to discourage you than to expect too much from yourself and your body at the start. Start slowly and build gradually. Watching your improvement will be a reward in itself. These are the government guidelines of physical activity:

- All adults aged nineteen and over should aim to be active daily, which means moving more and sitting less throughout the day.

- Moderate physical activity should add up to at least 150 minutes (2 hours and 30 minutes) to 300 minutes (5 hours) a week, which can be done as little as 10 minutes at a time. That is a total of about 22 to 45 minutes a day. Activities of daily living such as walking the dog, housework, and gardening count.

- If you prefer, you can opt for vigorous activity for 75 minutes (1 hour and 15 minutes) to 150 minutes (2 hours and 30 minutes) a week for maximum health benefits, which equals about 11 to 21 minutes a day.

- You can mix moderate and vigorous exercise during the week. one minute of vigorous intensity activity is about the same as two minutes of moderate intensity activity. You have to exercise half as much if your exercise is vigorous.

- You should do muscle-strengthening activities of moderate or greater intensity that involve all major muscle groups on two or more days a week.

- Older adults who are at risk of falls should incorporate physical activity to improve balance and coordination.

What Is Moderate Exercise, Anyway?

If you are not certain what the difference is between moderate and vigorous exercise, your body will tell you. Moderate exercise is not too taxing:

- Your breathing quickens, but you're not out of breath.
- You develop a light sweat after about 10 minutes of activity.
- You can carry on a conversation, but you cannot sing.

To give you an idea of what qualifies as moderate physical activity, I will list some examples:

Walking (2.5 mph)

Biking at light effort (10 to 12 mph)

Walking up stairs

Water aerobics

House cleaning—vacuuming, mopping, etc.

Tennis doubles

Water Aerobics

Gardening

Raking leaves

Washing a car

When Does Exercise Become Vigorous?

Vigorous intensity exercise feels challenging. Your activity is vigorous when:

- Your breathing is deep and rapid.
- You develop a sweat after only a few minutes of activity.
- You can't say more than a few words without pausing for breath.

The following list includes some vigorous activities to clarify the difference between moderate and vigorous activity:

Speed walking or walking uphill

Biking faster than 12 mph or uphill

Running or jogging

Strength training

Jumping rope

Singles tennis

Swimming laps

Shoveling snow

Cross country skiing

Dancing

One of the strategies of my program is to get you moving. As you will see in the pages that follow, you can add more activity to your life painlessly. The benefits of doing so are incalculable.

KEEP MOVING

You do not have to exhaust yourself for hours at the gym. Just take it slow and steady. If you are sedentary, you might begin by standing more during the day. No matter what you are doing, get up every twenty minutes or so and walk twenty feet, or just stand for two minutes. You can set the alarm on your phone to remind you to get up.

Adding more movement to your life does not have to be torture. I like to equate movement with recreation. An after-dinner walk, gardening, dancing, biking, hiking, yoga, tennis, or golf are all enjoyable ways to move more. Walking, swimming, and biking will help to reduce back pain. I consider this sort of recreational activity a moving meditation. Repetitive, consistent movement can alter your state of consciousness and create a feeling of tranquility and calm.

EASY WAYS TO ADD ACTIVITY TO YOUR LIFE

Stand or pace when you are on the phone.

Hide the remote.

Take a short walk every day after lunch and dinner.

Stop using drive-thrus.

Plant an herb garden or a perennial bed.

Sign up for a fitness class.

Dance while you do housework.

Stand on public transportation.

Fidget.

Walk to a co-worker's office instead of emailing.

Take up an atctive hobby—pole dancing, yoga, skiing, fencing, ballet, cycling, hiking.

Use your phone's pedometer or wear a fitness tracker.

Offer to watch a toddler.

Don't use the elevator or get off a floor or two earlier.

Join a sports league.

Walk or bike to work.

Don't waste TV time—use light weights for an arm workout or do stretches.

Do a plank during commercials.

Get off a stop early on public transportation and walk the rest of the way.

Waiting in line or in a doctor's office, do calve raises or stretches.

Meet friends for a walk rather than at a café or restaurant.

Get a standing desk, stationary bike, or treadmill.

You get the idea. There are countless ways to enjoy more movement.

Aerobic activity is critical for a healthy spine because it increases blood flow to the structures of your back. The deep breathing produced by aerobic activities improves the motion of the spinal joints, especially the facet joints, the spinal cord, and the nerve roots, and increases the flow and distribution of the cerebrospinal fluid (CSF). In addition, aerobic activity can decrease the swelling of problem joints and nerve roots. Aerobic exercise improves disc hydration and pumps more oxygen and nutrition to discs and joints to promote healing.

I do not recommend doing high-impact aerobics if you have back problems. The pounding and jarring movement will only aggravate your pain. You do not have to train for the marathon to benefit from exercise. Walking is great for your spine. It promotes spine joint mobility as well as nerve root movement and function. The more your facet joints and nerves move, the better you will feel. When you walk uphill, the joints of your spine are in a flexed open position, which might be helpful if your problem is nerve root tightness. Uphill walking can help patients with spinal stenosis because it opens up the spinal channel.

IF THE SHOE FITS

Shoe fit is important when you start to move more, especially for people who stand all day, including doctors, nurses, teachers, wait staff, and flight attendants. The average adult takes 4,000 to 18,000 steps a day, with men taking more steps than women. The fit of a shoe determines how forces are transmitted from the foot to the ground, which is known as the foot/ground interface or the person/ground interface.

Some people's feet have a more supinated position or roll outward, others have neutral rotation, and some have pronated feet that roll inward. The arches of the feet can be high, neutral, or flat. Most running and walking stores along with ski shops will provide a free assessment of the posture of your foot as you walk or run on a treadmill. They may create a personalized arch support for you that optimizes the strike of the foot in the foot/ground interface.

Shoes and sneakers come in a variety of support, softness, flexibility, and cushioning. I recommend starting with proper sizing, length, and width. Work with a footwear expert to determine the characteristics of your foot. Then try the shoe or sneaker on for comfort, cushioning, and feel. Improperly fitted shoes can be a direct cause of back pain. Reasonably lightweight and deeply cushioned, the sneaker helps them to walk again and to diminish the foot strike forces that can reverberate to the spine to cause back pain.

NOT ALL SURFACES ARE CREATED EQUAL

Walking on pavement leads to a firmer striking ground. The foot hits the hard pavement, and the forces are equally and oppositely returned to the foot. Hard concrete or pavement reverberates shock waves that oscillate through the body, which may lead to muscle spasms and neck and back pain.

Walking on soft dirt leads to a striking ground that gives way. The foot hits the soft ground, and the dirt moves, dissipating the striking forces. Less force is returned to the foot. Mechanically, soft dirt leads to less impact returned to the body. Soft dirt feels better, is less jarring, and may be the correct prescription for an older athlete or for a person who wishes to prolong their walking and running life.

WALK AWAY FROM PAIN

Walking is an easy way to add physical activity to your day. You can park your car far from the entrance to the supermarket, get off the bus a stop early and walk the rest of the way, go for a walk with a friend instead of sitting in a coffee shop—you can drink the coffee while you walk. It all adds up. You do not have to aim for 10,000 steps a day right from the start. If movement is not a normal part of your day, start out walking for five minutes and work up to walking for thirty minutes. The thirty minutes do not have to be consecutive. You can break up that time you spend walking any way you want.

Over time, you will feel positive changes that will motivate you to move more. You can take a walk outside and enjoy the sunshine and fresh air, or you could use a treadmill. To get optimum aerobic benefit and to protect your back, walking with proper form is important. Here are some tips:

- Keep your head up straight and focus on the horizon.

- Keep your shoulders relaxed without a forward slouch.

- Keep your stomach pulled in to support your spine.

- Avoid leaning forward as you walk.

- You do not have to take long strides—your stride should feel natural.

- Hold your arms close to your body with your elbows bent at a 90-degree angle. As you walk, keep your arms in front-to-back motion in pace with the stride of the opposite leg.

- Avoid clenching your hands or making tight fists. Your hands should be relaxed.

- Land gently on your heel and mid-foot with each step. Then roll to push off with your toes. Use the balls of your feet and toes to push forward with each step.

- If you opt for a treadmill, try to avoid holding on to the handrails. You should be walking slowly enough to avoid balance problems.

- Start out walking for 5 minutes and work up to walking for at least 30 minutes at least 3 or 4 times a week.

- Walk briskly but maintain enough breath to carry on a conversation.

20 ANYWHERE, ANYTIME STRETCHES

You don't have time to exercise? In answer to that common excuse, I have put together twenty stretches that can be done at your desk or just about anywhere. Most of the moves will probably go unnoticed by others around you.

There are many reasons why you should incorporate stretching into your daily activity. These simple moves will release muscle tension, help you to relax, improve your balance and awareness of your posture, increase the efficiency of your movement, and provide relief from pain and cramping.

There is not a set order for the twenty stretches, and there is no need to do all of them at once. As you learn to read where tension is building in your body, you will pick the tension-relieving stretch that makes you feel great.

Head Drop and Raise (Neck Flexion and Extension)

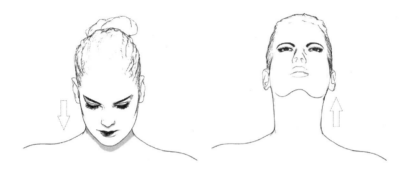

This stretch reduces tightness of the muscles in the front and back of the neck and increases flexibility. When you flex your neck forward, the upper muscles of your shoulders are targeted as well. When you bend your head back, you stretch your upper chest muscles, which need stretching if you are bent over a computer or tend to slouch.

- Sit comfortably in a chair with your feet flat on the floor and your neck in a neutral position right above your spine. Make sure your neck is not jutting forward or back.

- Straighten your spine and slowly lower your head forward with your chin close to your chest. Hold for 10 seconds.

- Slowly raise your head and tilt it back. You will be looking at the ceiling. Hold that position for 10 seconds.

- Return to your original position. Repeat 5 times.

Neck Tilts

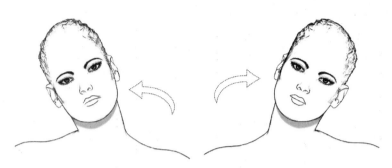

This movement will work the sides of your neck. The goal of these stretches is to make the muscles of your neck stronger and more limber. When properly stretched, the muscles will keep your neck upright and relaxed.

- Sitting with a straight back and your feet on the floor, slowly tilt your head to the right. Try to bring your ear as close to your shoulder as possible. Be sure not to raise your shoulders or force the movement. Hold for 10 seconds.

- Return your head to a neutral position. Tilt your head left to the other side. Hold 10 seconds. Repeat this stretch 5 times.

Neck Rotations

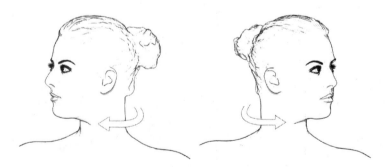

Rotating your neck will relieve neck pain and improve its range of motion.

- With a straight spine and your head erect, turn your head the right, chin high. Keep your shoulders relaxed. Hold for 10 seconds.

- Return your head to center, then turn your head to the left. Hold for 10 seconds.
- Return to center.
- Repeat 5 times.

Shoulder Shrugs

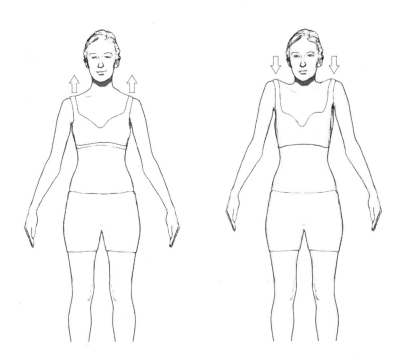

Shrugs build the strength of your shoulder, neck, and upper back muscles. Strengthening these muscles stabilizes your neck and upper back and reduces strain on your neck. It is a great stretch for posture improvement.

- Sit on the edge of your seat or stand with your knees slightly bent. Lift your chest and raise both shoulders up toward your ears. Hold for 5 seconds.
- Relax by dropping your shoulders down.
- Repeat 15 times.

Shoulder Rolls

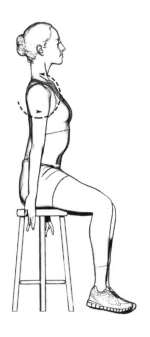 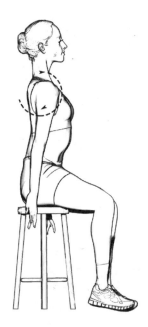

This stretch releases tension in the muscles of your neck, shoulders, and upper back. Shoulder Rolls help to develop better posture because the movement puts the body in a naturally correct posture position.

- Sit on the edge of your chair with your back straight and your head centered over your shoulders.

- Move your right shoulder back and up toward your chin. Roll your shoulder forward and down. Roll your shoulder 5 times.

- Repeat this with your left shoulder. Roll your shoulder 5 times.

- Switch to the opposite direction. Move your right shoulder forward and up toward your chin. Roll your shoulder back and down. Repeat 5 times.

- Repeat this on the left side. Repeat 5 times.

Chest Stretch

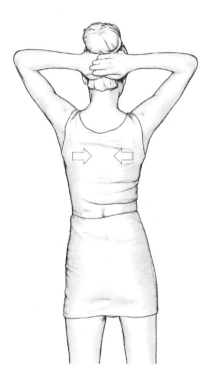

This exercise can be done sitting or standing. It improves posture by countering slouching. By stretching the muscles of the upper body, it relieves soreness and tightness in the chest and upper back.

- Place your hands on the back of your head with your elbows pointing to the sides of the room.

- Tilt your head back into your hands and open your chest.

- Squeeze your shoulder blades together and hold position for 20 seconds.

- Relax.

- Repeat 3 to 5 times.

Arm Across Chest Stretch

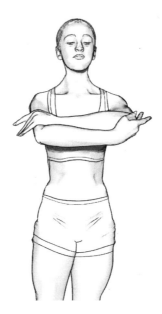

This stretch can be done while sitting or standing. It helps with upper body flexibility as it targets the shoulders and upper back.

- Raise your right arm in front of you to shoulder height, palm down.
- Bend your arm at the elbow, forearm parallel to the floor.
- Take your right elbow with your left hand and pull it gently across your chest.
- You will feel a stretch in your upper arm and shoulder on the right side.
- Hold for 20 seconds, then relax both arms.
- Repeat on your left side.
- Repeat 3 times on each side.

Arm Circles

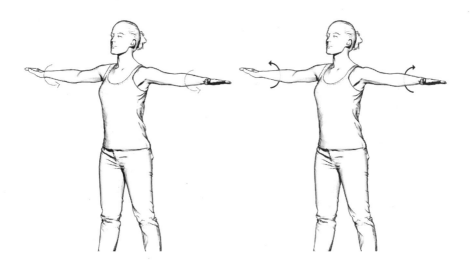

You can do this move sitting or standing. Arm Circles warm up shoulders, arms, chest, and back muscles, which is especially helpful if you have been sitting in one position too long. This movement relieves shoulder pain.

- Stand straight with feet shoulder width apart. Raise your arms to the sides parallel to the floor without bending your elbows. Your palms should be facing down.

- Slowly rotate your arms forward, making small circles about 5 inches in diameter. Do this for 1 minute. Drop your arms and relax.

- Repeat the exercise with your arms moving in the opposite direction, backward. Do this for 1 minute.

Arms Back Row

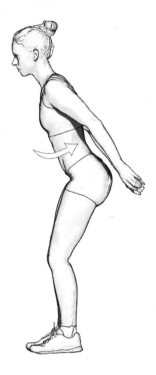

This is a simplified version of the classic straight arm back press. It targets your back muscles and your core. If you want to make this more challenging, you can hold a weight in each hand.

- Stand with your arms by your sides and your palms facing back. Engage your stomach muscles and sit back into a slight squat.

- Keeping your core engaged and your arms straight, slowly press your arms past your hips and hold for 5 seconds.

- Return to the starting position in a controlled motion. Avoid swinging your arms or bending your elbows.

- Repeat 12 to 15 times.

Overhead Shoulder Stretch

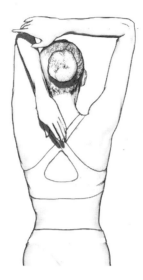

This triceps stretch will put your body into proper postural alignment. It energizes your shoulders, neck, and upper back.

- Stand with your shoulders back, chest out, and feet shoulder width apart.

- Raise your right arm overhead, bend your elbow, and place your hand behind your neck.

- Grasp your elbow with your other hand. Gently pull it behind your head.

- To increase the stretch, attempt to reach down between your shoulder blades and along your spine with the hand that is behind your head. Do not force the stretch.

- Hold the stretch for 10 seconds.

- Repeat the stretch on the other side.

Standing Backbend Stretch

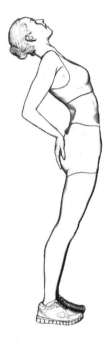

This stretch boosts the flexibility of the lower spine. The movement counters rounded, hunched shoulders. It stretches neck, shoulders, back, and core muscles. A backbend stretch opens up the front of the body, which helps your cardiovascular, digestive, and respiratory systems that are compressed when you hunch forward.

- Stand with your feet slightly apart. Place your hands on your lower back with your fingers interlaced, index fingers pointing down.

- Pull up your kneecaps and squeeze your thighs and buttocks.

- Press your hips forward and slowly arch your torso backward by rolling your shoulders and arching your lower spine as much as possible. Stretch your arms down. Keep your legs and buttocks engaged and strong.

- If your balance is good, you can drop your head back.

- Hold for 15 to 20 seconds.
- Inhale to lift your torso, followed by your head and neck to return to the starting position.
- Repeat the stretch 3 times.

Seated Forward Fold Stretch

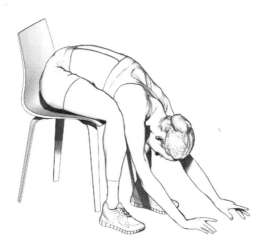

This is a great stretch to do if you have been sitting for hours in front of a computer screen. It reduces tension in your neck, shoulders, lower back, and hips. An added benefit: this stretch lowers blood pressure.

- Sit in a chair with your knees together and your feet flat on the floor.
- Take a deep breath. As you exhale, round your shoulders and bend forward one vertebra at a time.
- Let you head drop completely, and your arms fall by your side, hands touching your feet.
- Hold for 30 to 60 seconds before returning to starting position.

Seated Lateral Trunk Stretch

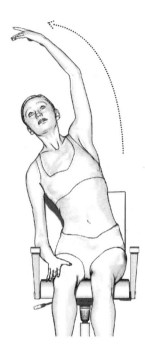

This stretch relaxes the muscles along the sides of your body and your spine, which relieves back and shoulder pain. Raising your arm overhead stretches the muscles of your shoulders and lower back.

- Sit in a chair with your feet flat on the floor.

- Raise your right arm over your head and place your left hand on your thigh for support.

- Slowly bend to the left until you feel a stretch along the right side of your torso.

- Hold the stretch for 15 to 20 seconds. Return slowly to center.

- Repeat the stretch with your left arm raised and lean to the right.

- Alternating sides, repeat the stretch up to 3 to 5 times.

Seated Twist

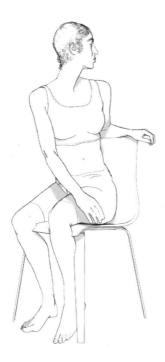

This yoga posture increases spinal flexibility. Though I have been recommending that you avoid twisting your spine, this position is static, and you do support your spine with your hands. It is relaxing and invigorating at the same time. The twist also promotes good digestion.

- Sit with your feet on the floor and your knees at a 90-degree angle. Move a bit forward in your seat, but not so far as to feel like the chair may tip forward or that you are unstable.

- As you inhale, sit up straight, lengthening your spine, and lift your arms overhead.

- As you exhale, turn gently to your right. Place your left hand on the outside of your right knee and your right hand on the chair behind you. Do not use your right hand to push you into a deeper twist. You do not want to use arm strength to twist your spine.

- Stay in the twist, inhale, and twist a little deeper as you exhale.

- Take 3 to 5 breaths before releasing the twist and repeating it on the other side.

- Stretch at least twice on each side.

Modified Downward Facing Dog

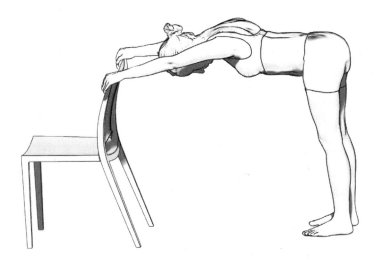

This yoga position elongates the upper and lower back and chest. By stretching the hamstrings, it increases the range of motion in the hips and relieves back pain.

- Stand about 2 or 3 feet in front of a stable chair with your feet about 18 inches apart.

- Raise your hands overhead.

- Slowly bend forward with a straight back until your hands are on the back of the chair. Keep your head aligned with your spine. Do not drop your head.

- Hold the position for 20 to 30 seconds or as long as you are enjoying the stretch.

Seated Pigeon Stretch

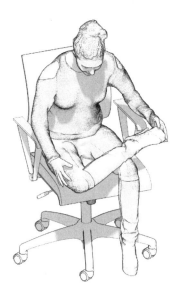

This pose works wonders on tight hips. While opening your hips, it increases the range of motion in the hips. The increased flexibility eases lower back pain. This is a preferred stretch for sciatica. Do not do this stretch if you have a total hip replacement, for fear of a dislocation.

- Sit forward on a chair so that you are not leaning back into the chair with your feet shoulder width apart.

- Rest your right ankle on your left knee or thigh. If it is painful, you can stretch out your left leg with your heel on the floor and rest your right ankle lower down on your left leg.

- Press your right knee down gently. If you feel a deep stretch while sitting erect, breathe into it.

- For a deeper stretch, lean forward from the hip with your spine long as far as you are comfortable.

- Stay in this position for 7 to 10 deep breaths.

- Repeat with your left leg on your right knee. One side will probably be tighter than the other. Hold the stretch longer on the tighter side.

Seated Leg Raiser

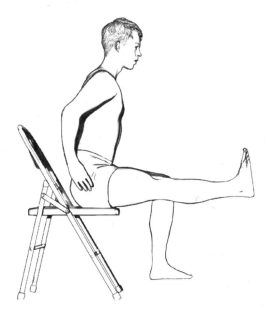

Though this movement might seem to work your abs, it actually targets your hip flexors. It helps to stabilize the pelvis and maintain proper hip movement. Begin by raising one leg at a time and build to raising both legs.

- While seated, lift one or both feet off the floor until your legs are straight in front of you.

- Lower your legs without letting your feet touch the floor.

- Repeat 15 times, alternating legs if you are raising them separately.

Seated Hamstring Stretch

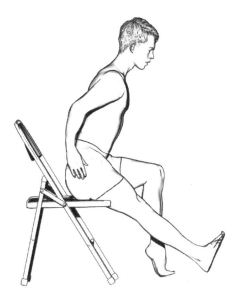

If you sit a lot, your hamstrings tighten. When your hamstrings are tight, the mobility of your pelvis is affected. Your pelvis rotates back, which subjects your lower back to more pressure. The resulting tilted position of the pelvis flattens the natural arch in your lower back. This stretch will help to prevent or fix that bad posture.

- Seated in a chair, straighten your right leg with your heel on the floor.

- Lean forward with your back straight and feel a stretch in your right hamstring.

- Hold the stretch for 20 to 30 seconds, then repeat with your left leg forward.

- Repeat 4 times for each leg.

Wall Squats

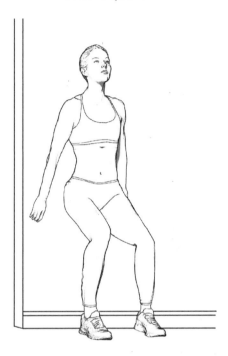

This is one of the best exercises you can do. Few exercises work as many muscles. Wall Squats work glutes, quads, and hamstrings, and build strength in the entire body. This exercise increases endurance, balance, and mobility.

- Stand with your back against the wall.

- Bend knees and slide your back down the wall until your thighs are parallel to the floor.

- Hold for at least 30 to 60 seconds. Try to hold as long as you can and gradually increase the length of your hold. Your legs will start to tremble.

- Keeping your back against the wall, rise gently by straightening your knees.

Standing Leg Curl

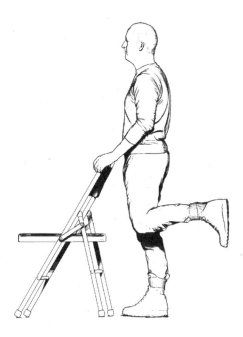

As the body ages, standing leg curls help prevent back pain by building the strength and flexibility of the hamstrings. The exercise improves balance as well, which is important as you get older.

- Put your hands on the back of a chair and stand with your feet shoulder width apart.

- Bend your right knee back at a 90-degree angle and slowly lift your right leg with your foot flexed. Aim your heel for the top of your right thigh.

- Lower your foot back down and repeat the curl with your left leg.

- Repeat 10 to 20 times on each leg.

These twenty moves will relieve tension in your muscles after a long time working at the computer, driving a long distance, or bingeing that show you missed. They will strengthen key muscles that support your back and improve your posture. For the best results, stretch whenever you feel uncomfortable. When you get up or change position every twenty minutes, do a stretch. Your back will thank you.

BEING A SPINE SURGEON PUTS ME AT RISK FOR SPINE PROBLEMS

As the author of our text neck study, I am happy to say that we helped the world lift its head up, but, as a surgeon, I risk developing text neck myself. Forward head posture (FHP) is a common problem for surgeons. We need to perform surgery with our hands without elevating our arms, and at the same time, we have to be able to observe closely the procedure we are performing. We can be on our feet for hours with our heads bent over or leaning in with our chins jutting. Surgeons have to pay special attention to the health of their spines.

To prepare for surgery, I make sure that I sleep well the night before. I start my day with a long, hot shower. I do stretches for my neck, shoulders, arms, and legs. I do not want tension in my muscles to distract me while I am operating. I find that stretching my hamstrings before surgery helps me to stay comfortable when I operate. Isometric pushes or a few push-ups, sit-ups, and lunges are my go-to exercises for strengthening. I try to stay adequately hydrated before, during, and after surgery.

Postural protection of my neck is critical as I perform surgery. The latest operating room equipment takes this into account. Today, operating room tables can be rotated, which reduces the need for surgeons to look down and diminishes the tilt of the head and neck. Surgical telescopes are now built at a downward angle, which minimizes surgeons' need to look down and risk straining their necks.

I use the Watch Your Back program myself to keep fit, flexible, calm, and strong. As you will see, I follow my own advice:

- I enjoy belly breathing and do my Count to Five belly breathing a hundred times a day.

- I regularly stretch my neck, back, hamstrings, quadriceps, Achilles tendons, and right and left shoulders.

- I rely on postural stretches to deeply open up my chest. The postural and hamstring stretches keep me in shape to perform surgery.

- For strength work I do sets of 10 push-ups, a few minutes of planking, sets of 10 sit-ups, sets of 25 squats, and sets of 10 lunges. I find deep, low squats particularly effective for charging me up.

- I run in place for aerobics: 30-second sets high knees (lifting knees to chest), 30-second sets mid-stance running (equal steps forward and backward), and 30-second sets of butt kicks (kicking feet to buttocks).

- Finally, I do one or two guided meditations from *Lift: Meditations to Boost Back Health* (see page 262 for more information).

My routine gives me the stamina, energy, and relaxation that enables me to perform complicated surgeries without experiencing muscle tension and exhaustion.

THE LIFE AQUATIC

Swimming and water exercise are ideal for alleviating back pain because they stabilize your spine and core. Strong back, abdominal, and hip muscles are key elements to maintaining a healthy spine. Since it is low impact, water exercise is especially good for older people. You can strengthen and condition these muscles safely in the water because there is no gravity. The buoyancy takes weight off your joints. Water offers firm resistance without impact.

Exercising in water is an efficient way to tone and strengthen. Water can have twelve times the resistance of air, which makes your muscles work harder. Consider any time you get in the pool extra credit.

Swimming laps is wonderful full-body exercise. The crawl, the breast-stroke, the side stroke, the back stroke work all the important muscle groups in your body. If swimming does not appeal to you, I recommend trying simple water aerobic exercises to strengthen your core and make you more flexible. The following six aquatic exercises are great conditioners:

Water Walking/Jogging

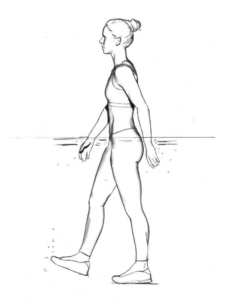

The resistance of the water makes muscles work harder, which strengthens them. Water walking is like power walking without impact on your knees, hips, and back. I was intrigued by a study of people with spinal stenosis that showed that their balance and muscle function improved after twelve weeks of water walking.

- Stand in waist or chest-high water with your weight evenly distributed on both feet. Take 10 to 20 steps forward. Remember to engage your stomach muscles and to keep your back straight.

- Jog gently in place for 30 seconds.
- Then take 10 to 20 steps backward.
- Continue back and forth for up to 5 minutes.
- To increase the intensity of the exercise and make it more challenging, simply move faster.

Side-Stepping

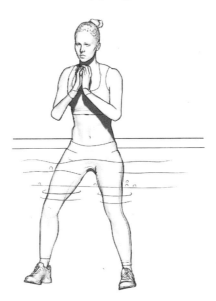

Moving side-to-side uses a different set of muscles from walking straight ahead. Lateral movement strengthens underused muscles, specifically the hip abductors and external rotators. By strengthening these muscles, you even the muscular balance in your hips, which is great for your lower back.

- Face the pool wall. Bend your knees slightly. Take sideways steps with your body and feet facing the pool wall.
- Take 10 to 20 steps in one direction and take 10 to 20 steps to return.
- Repeat twice in each direction.
- To increase the intensity, take bigger side steps or move more quickly.

One Leg Balance

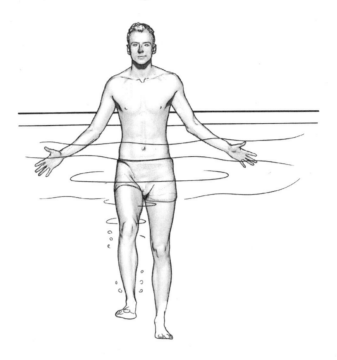

Balance is an important part of a healthy back. Doing a One Leg Balance in water works the entire lower part of your body—outer thighs, quads or front of thighs, groin, glutes, hip flexors, hamstrings, and calves. It does wonders for lower back pain. This balance exercise is especially good for seniors.

- Put all your weight on your right leg and raise your left leg 6 to 12 inches.

- Keep your hands under water, palms up, elbows slightly bent. If you feel unsteady, stand sideways and hold onto the wall.

- Hold the position for as long as you can comfortably. Repeat 4 or 5 times.

- Then perform the same exercise on the other side, standing on your left leg and raising your right.

- If you want a bigger challenge, try closing your eyes.

Knee-to-Chest

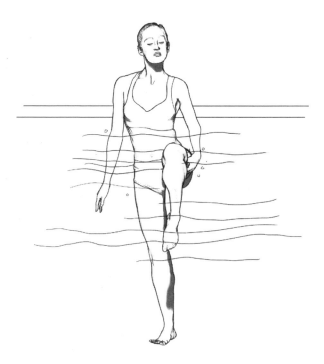

This exercise strengthens muscles in the leg, hip, and lower back. It restores flexibility to the lower back, increases joint flexibility, and reduces stiffness related to spinal stenosis.

- Stand with your left leg near the pool wall and your left hand on the side of the pool for balance if necessary.

- Put your weight on your left leg, keeping your left knee soft.

- Lift up your right leg with a bent knee. Slowly raise your knee as high as you can comfortably. You can support your right leg by holding that leg behind the knee with your right hand. Your goal is to bring your knee to your chest. Repeat 5 times.

- Reverse position with your right leg near the wall and your left knee bending toward your chest. Repeat 5 times on that side.

Hip Kicker

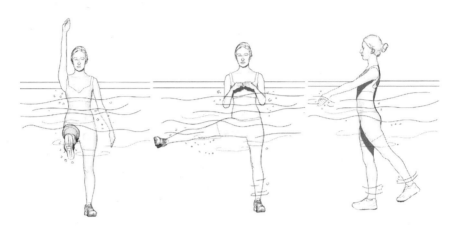

This is a range of motion exercise. When you lift your leg forward (flexion), you strengthen your hips. Moving to the side (lateral) works the abductors, the outside hip muscles, increasing stability and strength. Lifting your leg behind you (extension) helps to stabilize your back.

- Stand near the pool wall on the left side of your body for support.

- Slowly move and lift your right leg forward with a straight knee as if you are kicking. Keep your back straight. Do not buckle at the waist. Drop your right leg back to starting position.

- Then lift your straight right leg out to the side. Stay erect. Do not lean into or away from the lift. Return that leg to starting position.

- Finally lift your right leg straight behind you without arching your back. If you cannot keep your back erect with any of the three movements, you are lifting too high.

- Repeat the sequence with your left leg kicking.

- Repeat 10 times on each leg and build to 3 sets.

Superman

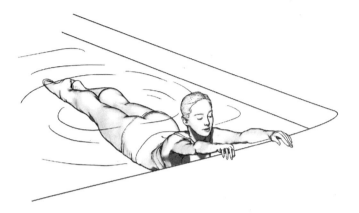

Flying like Superman as you are suspended in water strengthens your erector spinae muscles, a group of muscles and tendons, which run on the right and left of the spine from the sacrum to the skull. As their name indicates, they hold the spine erect. Doing Supermans helps to improve your posture.

- Stand facing the pool wall with your hands on the ledge of the pool.

- Slowly extend your body back with your legs straight. The idea is to look like Superman flying. Be sure not to hyperextend your back.

- Hold the position for 5 seconds, then bring your legs down.

- Repeat 5 to 10 times.

Now you have the know-how to reduce your back pain and stress by increasing your everyday activity and by gently stretching your muscles. Achieving these goals is easily within your reach. Do not be concerned about how you are going to do it all. The Watch Your Back program gives you a blueprint for structuring your day without overwhelming your routine. When you experience the physical and emotional improvements that result from taking action, you will grow to crave movement. Once you no longer feel bogged down, the thought of being sedentary will become disagreeable. I have seen this transformation in my patients so often. There is something liberating about choosing a path that shifts them from damaging habits and behavior to a way of life that promotes comprehensive healing. Integrating the strategies of my program into your life will do the same for you.

Chapter 8

Strategy 5:
Strong and Supple

Targeted exercise is an important part of the Watch Your Back program. In addition to the twenty stretches in the previous chapter, I have put together two workouts to strengthen your spine, make it more flexible, and reduce or prevent back pain. These exercises have an additional benefit. They will strengthen your core, which is essential for maintaining a healthy back.

I have designed the two workouts, each consisting of six exercises, to fit easily into your life. Each workout takes no more than ten minutes a day. No matter how busy you are, you can carve out ten minutes to exercise. Though Workout 2 is a bit more challenging than Workout 1, you can do them interchangeably. When you get bored with one workout, switch to the other.

I recommend incremental increases in repetitions so that you can intensify these workouts as you get stronger. You will find that the more you do, the more you can do. In movement, exercise, and life, there is always room for improvement. As your spine gets healthier, your back pain will dissolve. If you make these simple exercises a part of your daily routine, you will look and feel better. Eventually, you will barely remember life without exercise. When you experience the results of your efforts, you will be on your way to developing a fitness habit.

BREAKING THROUGH EXERCISE RESISTANCE

Karen, at fifty-eight, came to me complaining of terrible back pain, which she said was changing her life in negative ways. During her fifties, she began to put on weight and kept on gaining. She was convinced it was due to the hormonal changes of menopause. She had outgrown all her clothes and had resigned herself to wearing slacks with elastic waists. It was hard not to notice that she was suffering from what is called central obesity, the subject of my belly fat study.

I suggested that her expanded waistline was at the root of her back problems. I explained my study to her. As she gained weight around the middle of her body, the increased belly fat was exerting additional force on her lumbar spine. That extra force was straining her back muscles, which had to work hard to keep her spine aligned. I asked her about the level of movement and exercise in her life.

She grimaced, and said, "I used to be very active, I played tennis, took step classes, and jogged. When I began to put on weight, I was self-conscious about attending a class or going to a gym. Aside from being embarrassed about my body, I was finding it more difficult to exercise than I did in the past. I was so clumsy and out of shape, and then the pain made it impossible. I know that not exercising is not good for me, but I am so worried that my back will only get worse if I try."

I told her how important it was for her to move more. I was not expecting her to start working out at a gym. Just getting up and standing or moving around every hour for a couple of minutes was a good beginning. I explained that walking around the house, cooking, cleaning, and vacuuming counted as movement. To encourage her, I told her about a study that would give her hope. The study found that metabolic shifts could occur within a few hours of home activities such as cooking, cleaning, climbing up and down stairs, and doing laundry.

She began taking short walks around the neighborhood after lunch and dinner. She was moving so well she added gardening to her hobbies.

As she became more active, we discussed her diet. She said she was careful but confessed that she had a sweet tooth. She could not refuse a bowl of ice cream and had a habit of eating a handful of small cookies every day. I suggested she reduce the number of cookies she ate a day, and then reduce the number of days a week she indulged her habit, until the cookies became a rare treat. Though she did not eat ice cream every day, she could cut back her ice cream consumption in the same way.

"You mean that's all there is to it?" she asked.

Karen was surprised by the simplicity of the cookie subtraction scheme. She was used to going on major deprivation diets, on which she would lose weight and then gain it right back when she went off the diet. I explained that many of my patients use a version of the cookie subtraction scheme, whether it was gradually cutting back on beer, salty snacks, or cola. Of course, factors such as body metabolism and exercise have a big role in weight change. Karen was already on the right track with exercise.

To boost her metabolism, I encouraged her to drink a lot of water, to eat a salad per day, and to choose protein and complex carbohydrates over simple carbohydrates. Increasing the variety and quantity of the vegetables, which are complex carbohydrates, she consumed would help to reduce the inflammation that was causing her pain. Rather than starving herself, I advised her to have smart snacks every three to four hours to help reduce hunger.

I stressed the importance of getting enough high-quality sleep, which is when the body builds and restores itself. I recommended she aim for a power nap in the day and more than seven hours of sleep at night.

Karen began to lose two to three pounds a month. After a year, she was proud of her twenty-five-pound weight loss, had joined a gym, and had almost no back pain.

NO NEED FOR A HOME GYM

I recommend dedicating a place to be your workout space. Defining an exercise area makes it easier to be consistent. If you do not have to figure out where to work out each day and if the space is clear of clutter, you can get right to it without delays. The process becomes automatic. And you will not have to worry about knocking over a lamp or bumping your leg on a chair.

The twelve exercises do not require jumping, leaping, large movements, or equipment. I designed the workouts to be as uncomplicated as possible. All you need is a space the size of a yoga mat. You could exercise at the foot of your bed, in a little-used dining room, a garage, a basement, or any clear space. Just make sure you have enough room to lie down.

Choose a place without a lot of traffic. You want to be able to do your workout without interruptions. If the spot is noisy, you could listen to music, with earbuds if necessary. It is important that the area is well ventilated and bright. I suggest you have water within reach. Staying hydrated when you exercise is important.

That is all there is to setting yourself up for success.

THE WATCH YOUR BACK WORKOUTS

I suggest that you do not mix up the exercises of the two workouts. Do one or the other workout in its entirety because there is an intentional flow to the sequence for maximum benefit. Remember to do the exercises slowly and deliberately. Do not push yourself too hard. If you are uncomfortable at any point, you have reached your limit and have gone too far. If that happens, you have to dial it back. In time, your flexibility will increase as well as your strength. The number of reps you can do will go up. Rather than dreading exercise, you will come to enjoy making the workouts a part of your life. It will be a time, however short, when you can escape the demands of your life. Focusing your attention on your body during these workouts will help you to transcend daily concerns. The results you achieve through exercise will not disappoint you.

WORKOUT 1

Pelvic Tilt

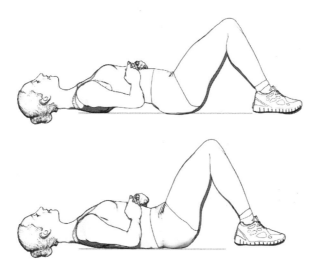

This is a stability exercise that promotes core control. If the abdominal muscles are not strong, your spine must work harder to keep your body in balance. When your core muscles are weak, your postural alignment is thrown off. Lumbar tilts are targeted to strengthen your lower abdominal muscles. This exercise will help to relieve pain and tightness in your lower back.

The exercise is recommended for the following spinal conditions: lumbar degenerative disc disease, spinal stenosis, lumbar spondylosis, spondylolisthesis, sciatica.

- Lie on your back with both knees bent and feet flat on the floor. Your arms can be resting by your sides, on your stomach, or behind your head, whatever is more comfortable.

- Keeping your shoulders pressed to the floor, tighten your abdominal muscles, and press the small of your back to the floor.

- Hold the contraction for 10 seconds, then release and take a few deep breaths to relax.

- Repeat 10 times.

The Hug (Knee-to-Chest Stretch)

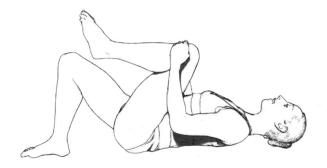

This stretch can stretch your lower back muscles and relax your hips, glutes, and thighs. The stretch helps to relieve pressure on spinal nerves by creating more space for those nerves as they exit the spine. The stretch works to relieve lower back pain.

- Lie on your back with your knees bent and your feet flat on the floor.

- Gently pull your right knee into your chest using both hands. You can either interlace your fingers under your knee or at the top of your shinbone, just below your knee. Avoid lifting your hips. You will feel a stretch in your lower back and a lengthening of your spine.

- Breathe deeply as you hold your knee against your chest for 30 to 60 seconds.

- Release your right knee and return your right leg to the floor.

- Repeat with your left leg.

- Repeat 3 times for each leg.

Cat-Cow Stretch

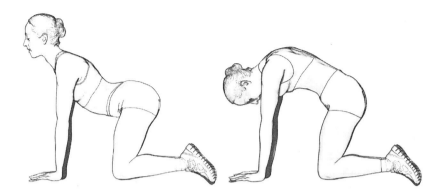

If you have ever done yoga, you will be familiar with this gentle exercise. The Cat-Cow movement helps to stretch the shoulders, neck, and chest as well as the muscles that run the length of your back. This exercise will increase your flexibility and ease tension in your lower back and core.

If being on your knees is painful, you can do this exercise in a chair with your feet flat on the floor and your hands on your knees.

- Come onto all fours in a tabletop position with your knees below your hips and your wrists below your shoulders. Take a deep breath.

- When you breathe out, arch your back by pulling your stomach in toward your spine. Your pelvis will tilt toward your ribs and your shoulder blades will draw away from each other. Let your head drop forward. This is the cat pose. Picture an angry, hissing cat.

- Hold for 5 to 10 seconds.

- When you breathe in, let your stomach drop toward the ground and raise your head. Do this slowly and deliberately. Your pelvis will fall forward, and your back will arch. This is the sway-backed cow pose.

- Hold for 5 to 10 seconds.

- Return to the starting position and repeat the stretch 10 to 20 times.

Bridge

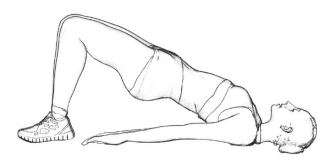

Bridges strengthen your gluteus maximus, or glutes, the large muscle of the buttocks. One of the most important muscles of the body, it supports the lower back. This exercise also works the muscles of the abdomen and the spinae erector, the muscles that run along the spine. The three muscle groups help you to hold an upright posture when you sit or stand.

- Lie on the floor with your knees bent, feet flat on the floor, hip-width apart. Pull your feet as close as you can to your buttocks. Keep your arms by your sides.

- While squeezing your buttocks, raise your pelvis toward the ceiling. Roll your torso upward until your back is off the ground. Your shoulders will be supporting your weight. Your body should form a straight line from your shoulders to your knees.

- Continue to squeeze your buttocks and hold for 5 seconds.

- Gently lower your torso one vertebra at a time until your back is flat on the floor.

- Take two deep breaths and repeat 7 to 12 times. Gradually build up to 3 sets.

Hamstring Stretch with Towel

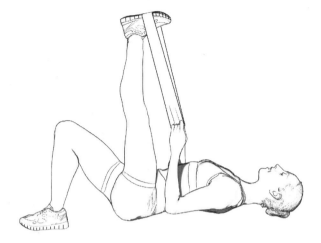

Your hamstring muscles run from the back of each thigh from the hip to the back of the knee. When you spend hours sitting with your knees bent at a desk all day or a lot of time driving, your hamstrings remain in a shortened position. The glutes need to move to stay healthy. Sitting too much causes a chain reaction: the hip flexor muscles in the front of each hip contract and tighten and tell the nerves to inhibit or turn off the glutes, the muscles that provide the opposite motion. Weak glutes then force the hamstrings to pick up the slack and do more of the glutes' job. But hamstrings also can become tight from too much sitting. It is a double whammy. When tight hamstrings are forced to work overtime, they are vulnerable to tears and strains.

This stretch will lengthen your hamstrings. If you can reduce tension in your hamstring muscles, you will reduce the stress you feel in your lower back.

- Lie on the floor with your left knee bent and your left foot flat on the floor.

- Wrap a towel or an exercise band behind your right knee, calf, or around your instep, depending on how flexible you are, and hold on to the ends.

- Keeping your stomach muscles tight, use the towel to lift your straight or slightly bent right leg until you feel a gentle stretch in the back of your right thigh. Hold for 15 to 30 seconds, then lower the right leg to the floor.

- Repeat 3 times per side, alternating your legs.

Cobra

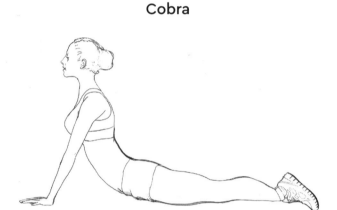

This yoga pose involves active back bending. If you experience mid-back pain, you may not be able to go very far at first. Do not push the stretch beyond what is comfortable. Bending back increases flexibility, helps to stretch your chest, and strengthens the muscles of your spine.

- Lie face down on the floor with your legs extended behind you, the tops of your feet resting on the floor.

- Place your hands under your shoulders with your fingers pointing forward. Bend your elbows and hold your arms close to your body.

- Push your legs and feet into the floor by engaging your buttocks and leg muscles. Doing this will support your lower back while your spine extends and your chest lifts.

- Breathe out. Push up slowly, using your arms to arch your back. Lift your head and then your chest from the floor.

- Try to bend back more by straightening your arms and lifting your chest farther from the floor. Your head should be aligned with your spine. Only go as far as is comfortable. Your flexibility should increase in time.

- Hold the position for 20 to 30 seconds. Gently return to the floor and repeat the stretch 3 or 4 times.

WORKOUT 2

Corner Stretch

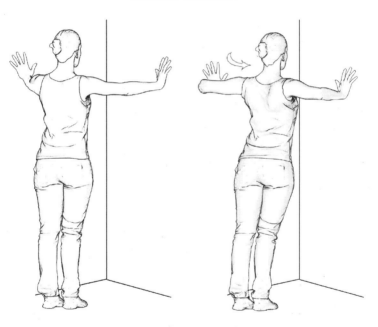

This stretch improves flexibility of your chest, arms, and shoulders. The Corner Stretch is great for your posture because it increases the strength of your upper back and opens your chest, a fix for hunched shoulders. By relieving tension in the neck and shoulders, the stretch alleviates neck pain.

- Stand facing a corner of the room with your feet together about 2 feet from the corner.

- Place a hand on each wall with your elbows slightly below shoulder height.

- Lean forward until you feel the stretch across your chest and shoulders. If you feel any pain, reduce the stretch by not leaning in as far.

- Hold the stretch from 30 to 60 seconds.

- Repeat 5 times.

Lying Lateral Leg Lifts

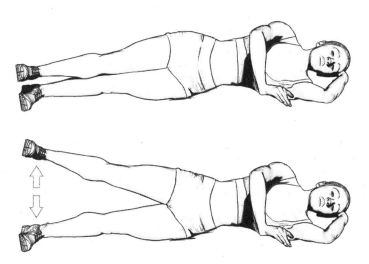

This exercise works your hip abductor muscles, which support your pelvis and can help to reduce strain on your back. It is important to keep your hip abductors strong because they help you to maintain balance and mobility. Lying Lateral Leg Lifts also work your glutes. Strong glutes contribute to stabilization of the knees, hips, and lower back.

- Lie on one side with your lower arm on the floor and your upper hand in front of your body. You can bend the elbow of your lower arm and rest your head in your hand or lie flat and with your head on your arm. Keep your legs together, your lower leg slightly bent.

- Tighten your stomach to engage your core muscles.

- Keeping your top leg straight and extended, slowly lift it about 18 inches.
- Hold that position for 10 seconds, then slowly lower your leg.
- Repeat 10 times.
- Turn onto the other side of your body and repeat, using your other leg.
- Work up to 3 sets.

Plank

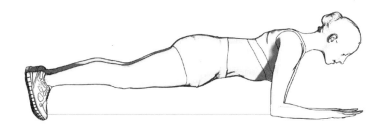

Planks are a super exercise with many benefits. This simple exercise engages all the muscle groups in your core to help support your back. Planks do not put pressure on your spine. In fact, doing Planks reduces back pain by strengthening the muscles supporting your back. This exercise improves posture, ensuring that your back is properly aligned. And if that isn't enough, your overall balance and flexibility will improve.

- Begin on your stomach, face down.
- Place your hands directly under your shoulders. Your fingers pointing forward.
- As you straighten your arms, ground your toes into the floor and squeeze your buttocks to stabilize your body.
- Keep your torso straight and rigid and your body in a straight line from ears to toes without sagging or bending.
- You should be looking at a spot on the floor about a foot beyond

your hands with your head relaxed. Your head should be in line with your back.

- Inhale and exhale slowly and steadily.

- Hold your position for as long as you can. You may start to tremble, which means you are working your muscles.

Modified Plank

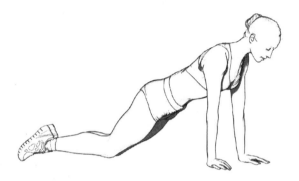

If you have trouble maintaining your Plank, try doing the exercise from bent knees, which is called a Modified Plank.

- Lie on the floor with your hands flat on the floor under your shoulders.

- Keeping your core engaged and your knees on the floor, slowly straighten your arms, raising yourself upward until your body is in a straight line from your knees to your head.

- Hold this Modified Plank for as long as you can, building to 1 minute. If you can hold your knee Plank for a minute, you are ready to graduate to a full Plank.

Supine Trunk Rotation

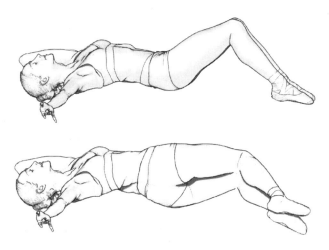

The trunk rotation stretch can help to relieve tension in your lower back. It works your core muscles, including your abs, back muscles, and the muscles in your pelvis. Building trunk stability and control is critical in easing lower back pain.

I am giving you a beginner's exercise to start with. As you get stronger, you can advance to a more challenging version of this stretch.

- Lie on your back with your knees bent, your feet flat on the floor, and your arms outstretched.

- Brace your stomach muscles, which will stabilize your lumbar spine.

- Slowly roll your knees to the right side while you press your shoulders and arms to the floor. Keep your knees together. Your upper body should stay firm against the floor. Do not force the rotation. This is not a big movement. Control is what is important.

- Hold the rotated position for 10 seconds and then slowly rotate your knees to the starting position.

- Rotate your knees to the left side and hold for 10 seconds.

- Repeat 5 to 10 times on each side.

Modified Trunk Rotation

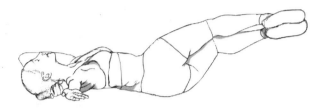

If you feel ready to progress, try a Modified Trunk Rotation by raising your feet. Doing this exercise with lifted feet increases resistance and requires a deeper abdominal brace. The rotation increases flexibility in the lower back and hips. It also improves flexion, extension, and rotation of the spine.

- Lie on your back with your arms extended. Bring your knees up toward your chest until your calves are parallel to the floor.

- Proceed to rotate your lower body as you did in the previous version of the exercise.

Bird Dog

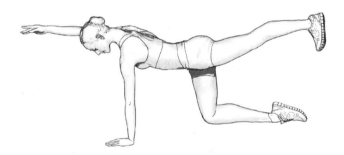

This core exercise improves spinal stability, encourages a neutral spine, and relieves lower back pain. Bird Dogs strengthen your core, hips, and back muscles, which contributes to correct movement and stability of the whole body. It promotes good posture and increases the range of motion of the lower back.

- Begin on all fours in the tabletop position with your knees hip-width apart and your hands shoulder-width apart.

- Engage your abdominal muscles to maintain a neutral spine and keep your back from sagging. Draw your shoulder blades together and down from your ears.

- It's a good idea to begin by practicing the movement. Lift one hand and the opposite knee just an inch off the floor and balance on the other hand and knee. Keep your weight centered. When you feel stable, you are ready to move to a full range of motion.

- Slowly raise your right arm and your left leg. Make sure to keep your shoulders and hips parallel to the floor. Do not rotate your pelvis. Avoid lifting your leg too high or allowing your spine to curve past its natural position. Avoid letting your chest sink to the floor. Hold the position for 10 seconds.

- Repeat 5 to 20 times.

- Return to the starting position and then repeat the exercise on the other side—raising the left arm and the right leg.

- Repeat 5 to 20 times.

Child's Pose

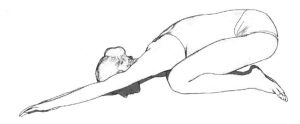

This restful yoga position relieves pain all along your spine, neck, and shoulders. As your trunk rests over your knees your spine will elongate passively. This position relaxes tight lower back muscles, promotes blood circulation along the spine, and increases flexibility.

- With your hands and knees on the ground, sink back and rest your hips on your heels or as close as you can get without straining.

- Fold forward by hinging at your hips. Walk your hands out in front of or alongside your body with your palms facing down.
- Rest your stomach on your thighs.
- Breathe deeply and focus on relaxing areas of tightness.
- Hold the position for up to 1 minute.
- Use your hands to return to an upright position.

Now that you are moving to ease your pain, it is time to consider how you are fueling that movement. Instead of feeding the fire of inflammation, what you eat can subdue the condition that is at the root of your pain.

Chapter 9

Strategy 6:
The Pain-Killing Diet

You can reduce your back problems and chronic pain by eating a balanced, anti-inflammatory diet, which includes vitamins and nutrients to nourish the bones, muscles, discs, and other spine structures. The food you eat can manage and prevent inflammation, or it can inflame your body. Chronic inflammation is at the root of most chronic pain, and what you eat affects the condition. You can choose to eat a pain-killing diet, which will improve your overall health.

Though inflammation has become associated with pain and disease, inflammation is not all harmful. It is a physical response that protects your health. If you are injured or have an infection, your body signals the immune system to send white blood cells to the affected area to repair the injury or fight the disease. Once the job is done, the inflammatory response subsides. When your stress levels are high, the "fight-or-flight" response turns on your immune system's inflammation response. Psychological distress can cause your body to remain in crisis mode. The turned-on response leads to chronic, low-grade inflammation, which can damage healthy cells and cause pain in muscles, tissues, and joints. A constant state of low-grade inflammation can lead to a number of serious diseases, including cancer, heart disease, diabetes, arthritis, depression, and Alzheimer's. Reducing inflammation in your body will not only quiet your back pain but can also prevent you from developing significant illnesses.

A good diet supports your immune system for optimal function, but a poor diet can activate your immune system and contribute to chronic, low-grade inflammation. Obviously, you want to eat foods that will help to regulate your immune system and to avoid foods that will inflame your body. Avoiding highly processed food and opting for fresh, whole food is the keystone for a pain-killing diet.

PROCESSED FOODS AND YOUR PAIN

If you want to ease chronic pain, you must edit what you eat. Eating food that is alive will make all the difference. Most of the packaged foods on the shelves of the grocery store probably have had the life processed out of them. If food is canned, jarred, bagged, or boxed with a long list of ingredients on the label, including many you cannot pronounce, consider it processed. The whole food has been stripped of nutrients during processing, then "enriched" with synthetic vitamins and minerals. Fiber is pulverized. Artificial chemicals are added to make food last longer and look better. Artificial flavor is an added chemical cocktail. Many of these chemicals promote inflammation.

A study reported in *Time* found that 60 percent of an American's daily calories come from "ultra-processed" food, defined as foods that contain ingredients such as flavors, colors, sweeteners and hydrogenated oils, emulsifiers, and other additives that you would not use to cook in your own kitchen. The study also noted that processed food is the main source of added sugar in the U.S. diet.

Sugar Fuels Inflammation

A diet high in sugar can lead to chronic, systemic inflammation. Sugar stimulates the production of free fatty acids in the liver. When the body digests these free fatty acids, the resulting compounds can trigger inflammation. I have to repeat that most forms of joint pain and muscle aches involve inflammation. Even if the pain is the result of a trauma, symptoms may be exacerbated and prolonged by eating foods high in sugar.

Sweetened drinks are among the worst sources of added sugar. The brain reacts when you eat sugar-rich foods because they have bulk. But with sugary drinks, which have no bulk, your body does not register the calories. You end up consuming more because the drink does not fill you up.

COLA CRISIS

A patient, Bob, came to me about his chronic back pain, which he told me made it difficult for him to be normally active. As far as he was concerned, exercise was out of the question. At five feet ten inches, he weighed more than three hundred pounds. Seeing that he was overweight, I started a conversation about his condition. I told him that his weight had a lot to do with his chronic back problems.

When I asked him how long he had been seriously overweight, he said he had begun to put on weight ten years earlier, that his weight had crept up at a rate of ten to fifteen pounds a year. We discussed his eating habits. He mentioned that he had gradually increased the amount of cola he was drinking. He was up to four two-liter bottles a day. That is a daily excess of 3,200 calories on top of what he was already eating. What had driven up his weight was obvious.

I introduced him to the Watch Your Back program and suggested ways he could move more. We blocked out a plan for reducing his cola intake. His weight loss did not happen overnight, but as he changed his eating habits and added movement to his day, he began dropping pounds.

His belief that he could meet his goal fueled his determination. As his weight went down, he embraced the strategies of the Watch Your Back program. He discovered he had so much more energy once he started moving. Though he had a way to go with his weight, within four months his pain significantly diminished.

Manufacturers add more refined sugar to food during processing, along with salt and bad fats. Two hundred years ago, the average American ate only two pounds of sugar a year. In 1970, that number went up to 123 pounds of sugar a year. Today, the average American consumes almost 152 pounds of sugar in a year. This is equal to consuming three pounds or six cups of sugar in a week. The rise in sugar consumption parallels the increased availability of convenience foods. No one is spooning out that much sugar. Most of it is hidden in processed food.

Overall, processed foods contain five times more sugar than unprocessed or minimally processed choices such as meats, fresh fruits or vegetables, whole grains, and milk.

The American Heart Association has published recommendations for sugar intake:

- Men should consume no more than 9 teaspoons (36 grams or 150 calories) of added sugar per day.

- Women should consume no more than 6 teaspoons (25 grams or 100 calories) per day.

To put these numbers in perspective, one twelve-ounce can of soda contains eight teaspoons (32 grams) of added sugar or 140 calories. One can of soda could max out your sugar intake for the day.

Simple Carbs vs. Complex Carbs

Most highly processed foods are made from refined ingredients like white flour. The highly refined simple carbohydrates found in processed foods are simple sugars, with nutrients such as vitamins and minerals removed. Candy, cookies, crackers, soda, sports drinks, "white food" such as bread, rolls, pasta, and white rice are loaded with simple sugars and starch. The problem with simple carbohydrates is that they are digested easily, causing your blood sugar to spike. Complex carbohydrates, brown rice, whole grains, beans, and most vegetables, for example, are starches combined with fiber. Complex carbs take longer to digest, which provides a steady, even stream of energy and keeps you feeling full longer.

I know that processed food is a broad category. To be more specific, I want to give you some general guidelines for food that can raise inflammation levels in your body:

Sugary Drinks: soda, fruit juices, energy drinks, sports drinks, sweet tea, sweetened specialty coffee drinks

Refined Carbohydrates: white bread, pasta, white rice, crackers, flour tortillas, biscuits, croissants

Fried Foods: french fries, fried onions, donuts, fried chicken, fried mozzarella sticks, egg rolls

Processed Meats: bacon, salami, hot dogs, smoked meat, pepperoni, beef jerky

Junk Food: fast food, convenience frozen meals, potato chips, pretzels, cheese doodles

Breakfast Foods: granola, breakfast cereals, cereal bars, pop tarts, muffins, bagels

Diet foods: low-fat yogurts, low-fat peanut butter, low-fat sauces, low-fat salad dressings, artificial sweeteners, low-calorie soda, low-carb anything

Canned Goods: baked beans, canned vegetables, canned fruit, some canned soups

Desserts: Candy bars, cookies, pastries, cakes, donuts, pies, tarts, ice cream, puddings, custards, ice pops

Trans Fats: shortening, partially hydrogenated vegetable oil, margarine

CAFFEINE AND JUNK FOOD

Edward, a fifty-four-year-old long-haul, big-rig driver, complained of severe back pain, especially after more than eight hours behind the wheel. Weighing 260 pounds at six feet tall, he was obese. To add to his problems, Ed had smoked a pack of cigarettes a day for twenty-five years. He was very worried about the increased frequency of near-miss accidents he was having on the road. He told me that leaving the job he had been doing for his entire adult life was not a possibility.

His MRI and X-rays showed advanced degenerative discs

of the two bottommost levels, L4-L5 and L5-S1. There was no significant compression of the spinal sac, the sheath that carries the spinal cord, nerves, and spinal fluid. I said that I would do my best to help him but warned that the solution to his back problems might take at least six months. He was more than happy to tackle his problems. For him, six months was nothing compared to the decades of discomfort he had suffered.

I gave him a new perspective on his smoking by informing him that he had smoked 9,125 packs of cigarettes over time, and that is a lot of tar in his lungs. Edward confessed that his cigarette smoking was worse than he had said. He often smoked two packs a day. He had known for some time that smoking was a habit he had to break. He claimed that his wife would not let him forget it. To help him quit smoking, we decided that his medical doctor should prescribe nicotine gum.

He was committed to changing. We moved on to his weight. He said it was hard to eat well on the road. He consumed a lot of junk food at truck stops and always kept a bag of sweet and salty snacks in the rig. He told me that he drank caffeinated drinks all day to perk him up because his energy was low. We considered a path to weight loss. We decided on a plan for him. I recommended cutting 500 calories per day = 3,500 calories per week to lose one pound a week, translating to fifty pounds in a year. If he aimed to lose 1/2 pound a week for two years, his fifty-pound loss would get him to his target weight. Looking at weight loss from this perspective made getting to a healthy weight seem less daunting and achievable. Edward promised to make better choices in eating and drinking on the road. He knew what he had to do.

His sleep habits were deplorable, and all the caffeinated beverages did not help. He told me that he slept about four hours a night on the road. He explained how hard it was to get restful sleep. "Many times, when you're sleeping at a truck stop, a truck pulls in and makes lots of noise with the hydraulic brakes.

I can't sleep through that."

We set the goal of getting six hours of sleep a night. He agreed to have a nap after lunch in the middle of the day. Edward came up with the idea of creating a sleeping chamber at home to help him catch up on his sleep. He aimed to get ten to twelve hours of sound sleep a night at home to make up for the sleep deficit he built up on the road.

Moving on, I told him that paying attention to his posture while driving could make a big difference in his comfort level. First, he agreed to stop and stretch twice a day. I explained that proper posture in his truck involved sitting tall, with lumbar support or a rolled-up towel behind his back and his feet resting on the floor or pedals. I suggested that he keep both arms on the armrests and both hands on the wheel when he was driving. The good news was that his seat had hydraulic shock absorption, which saved his spine every time he drove over a bump in the road.

I gave him an abdominal binder and a standard lumbar support brace to use when he needed extra support for his lower back.

A year later and forty pounds lighter, Edward was a different person. It was easy to see that he had been following my advice. Ed was consuming fewer caffeinated drinks and continued to chew nicotine gum. He cut his smoking to a half pack a day. Though he was not using the lumbar support brace, he loves his abdominal binder, which occasionally provides "just the right amount of support" when he needs it.

He was proud of all he had managed to accomplish. For the most part, he was now pain free. From time to time, Ed reported flare-ups, though nowhere as bad as before. Edward's good feelings spread to every aspect of his life. I was happy to see that he had committed to turning his life around.

NOT ALL FATS ARE CREATED EQUAL

Fats have a bad reputation, but the truth is that your body needs fat as a source of energy. Fat helps your body absorb some vitamins and minerals. It is necessary to build cell membranes and to sheath nerves. You have probably heard that industrially made trans fats are bad for you, monounsaturated and polyunsaturated fats are good for you, and saturated fats fall somewhere in between.

Trans fat is made from a process called hydrogenation, which turns healthy oils into solids. Trans fats have been banned in the United States because they have been found unsafe for human consumption. Trans fats used to be found in margarines and vegetable shortening. Food manufacturers learned how to make partially hydrogenated vegetable oils, now used in everything from cookies to fast food and french fries. The new version of trans fats, partially hydrogenated vegetable oils, creates inflammation.

Saturated fats are solid at room temperature. This type of fat is found in red meat, whole milk dairy foods, and many commercially prepared foods and baked goods. Not only are these bad for your cholesterol, but saturated fats also short-circuit your immune cells and trigger inflammation.

Good fats are found in vegetables, nuts, seeds, and fish. They are liquid at room temperature. Monosaturated fats are found in olive oil, peanut oil, canola oil, avocados, and most nuts. There are two main types of polyunsaturated fats, omega-3 fatty acids and omega-6 fatty acids. Omega-3s, found in fatty fish, walnuts, canola oil, and unhydrogenated soybean oil, are good for your health. Omega-6 fatty acids are found in safflower, soybean, sunflower, walnut, and corn oil. Omega-6 fats used to be thought to increase inflammation, but that evaluation has changed. The body can convert the most common omega-6 fat, linolenic acid, into fatty acid called arachidonic acid. Arachidonic acid is a building block for molecules that can promote inflammation. Recent research has shown that the body also converts arachidonic acid into molecules that calm inflammation. With that in mind, omega-3s seem a better bet.

EAT TO FIGHT INFLAMMATION

Though what you eat can contribute to chronic inflammation in your body, the good news is that your diet is one of the best ways to reduce inflammation and the pain that accompanies it. Your diet can help to support your immune system so that it turns on and off as it should, which prevents persistent, low-grade inflammation.

The Mediterranean diet is the best way to eat to get inflammation and pain under control. The foundation of this way of eating is built on plant-based foods, such as whole grains, vegetables, legumes, fruits, nuts, seeds, herbs, and spices. Olive oil is the primary source of added fat. Fish, seafood, dairy, and poultry are eaten in moderation. Red meat and sweets are rarely consumed.

My recommendations for a pain-killing diet are straightforward:

- Cut down on processed foods. You know how sugar, trans fats, and additives trigger inflammation.

- Build meals around vegetables and fruits. Emphasizing plant-based foods in your diet automatically increases your supply of antioxidants and phytochemicals that function as anti-inflammatory agents. Aim for at least five servings of vegetables, beans, and fruits a day.

- A good piece of advice is to "eat the rainbow." Fruits, vegetables, and beans come in a range of colors—red, orange, yellow, green, blue, and purple—and their rich colors serve a nutritional purpose. By eating fruits and vegetables in a rainbow of colors, you will get a variety of important vitamins and nutrients that will help to combat inflammation.

- Forget white bread, pasta, and rice. Go for whole grain products instead. Highly refined grains, used in white bread, for example, raise your blood sugar levels and contribute to inflammation. Experiment with brown rice, barley, bulgur, and quinoa instead of white rice.

- Eat fish at least twice a week. Focus on those with healthy omega-3 fatty acids, like salmon and mackerel (see page 195 for more choices).

- Use extra virgin olive oil instead of butter or other vegetable oils in preparing food. Olive oil is rich in monounsaturated oleic acid, which has been shown to reduce inflammatory markers. It contains vitamins E and K and other antioxidants. If you are cooking at high temperatures, substitute extra virgin coconut oil.

- Limit red meats, which are high in saturated fat and known to cause inflammation. Research findings are mixed, but a diet high in red meat has been found to make rheumatoid arthritis symptoms worse.

- Use spices liberally. Not only will your food be more delicious, but many spices prevent or reduce inflammation, among them cayenne, cinnamon, ginger, and turmeric.

- Serve fresh fruit for dessert. Skip the sugar-laden "treats" that will aggravate your pain.

- Limit alcohol consumption. Recent research suggests that alcohol causes inflammation in the intestines and impairs the body's ability to regulate that inflammation, which results in systemic inflammation.

STAY HYDRATED

Drinking water is necessary for your body to function optimally, but you probably do not think about how hydration affects your back. Research on astronauts has shown that the spaces between vertebral bodies change with the time of day and hydration levels. Other studies have shown that when we stand and our spine is vertical, gravity works on the spine, and the discs become compressed. Fluid is squeezed out. Over the course of the day, the spaces between the discs diminish, the curvature of the spine changes, and spinal flexibility is decreased. When you are horizontal during sleep and the pressure of gravity is removed, the hard discs rehydrate and swell, recovering the proper space between vertebrae.

A general recommendation for hydration is to drink eight eight-ounce glasses of water a day. Another calculation is to drink from one-half ounce to one ounce of water for each pound of your body weight daily. For example, if you weigh 170 pounds, you should drink 85 to 170 ounces of water a day, which converts to about eleven cups to twenty-one cups a day. The amount of water you need is affected by hot or cold weather, dry climate, high altitude, alcohol consumption, exercise, pregnancy, and sickness.

30 INFLAMMATION EXTINGUISHERS

Some foods are natural inflammation busters, packed with inflammation-fighting nutrients. Consuming more of these foods can help to reduce chronic inflammation and, even better, regulate inflammation by turning off the process before systemic inflammation can occur. I have compiled a list of thirty foods that have been scientifically proven to reduce inflammation and to prevent serious disease. Make certain to add these powerful foods to your diet. When inflammation levels are reduced, pain is as well. Consuming these superfoods on a regular basis can help to eliminate your back and neck pain and replace the need for anti-inflammatory drugs.

These thirty foods contain potent pain-killing nutrients. Rather than simply listing the foods, I have identified the healing nutrients in each. I want you to know how superfoods fight inflammation to inspire you to increase the amount of these foods in your diet. The overview that follows defines terms that appear in the nutritional information.

Omega-3 fatty acids, namely EPA and DHA, found in abundance in extra virgin olive oil, are very powerful anti-inflammatory agents. Vitamins C, A, and E in olive oil work to eliminate damaging free radicals. Minerals help to absorb nutrients and to flush out toxins that can cause inflammation. Fiber helps to break down food and keep the gut healthy.

Plant-based foods contain phytochemicals and phytonutrients known to combat inflammation. Polyphenols in plants protect them from UV rays and infection. As micronutrients in the food you eat, they protect your body by lowering inflammation and preventing disease.

Antioxidants neutralize free radicals, which damage cells. Free radical damage translates to inflammation on a cellular level. By attacking free radicals, antioxidants reduce inflammation. Many vitamins, polyphenols, and phytonutrients act as antioxidants.

Flavonoids, a large group of phytonutrients, have potent antioxidant and anti-inflammatory properties. I identify the flavonoids found in specific foods on the list, among them anthocyanins, quercetin, catechins, resveratrol, and kaempferol. Carotenoids, pigments that give plants red, orange, and yellow coloration, act as anti-inflammatory antioxidants. The carotenoids include alpha-carotene, beta-carotene, lutein, and lycopene.

With that brief nutritional review, you will be able to see how these superfoods fight inflammation.

1. **Almonds and Other Nuts**: Almonds, hazelnuts, peanuts, pecans, pistachios, and walnuts contain high amounts of fiber, calcium, magnesium, zinc, vitamin E, and omega-3 fats, which all have anti-inflammatory effects. Walnut skins have anti-inflammatory phenolic acids, flavonoids, and tannins.

2. **Avocados**: Rich in anti-inflammatory monounsaturated fats. They contain potassium and magnesium, which flush out toxins that cause inflammation. The antioxidants found in avocados, carotenoids and tocopherols, are found in vitamin E.

3. **Beans and Legumes**: Black beans, chickpeas, lentils, pinto beans, red beans, and black-eyed peas are great for you. Legumes are the seeds of plants that include beans, lentils, soybeans, peas, and peanuts. Beans and legumes are powerful anti-inflammatory foods because they are bursting with antioxidants and phytonutrients as well as being one of the richest sources of fiber on the planet. They are also an incredibly nutrient-dense

food full of vitamins and minerals, including B vitamins, calcium, magnesium, iron, zinc, and potassium.

They are exceptionally healthy foods for humans and animals, with the bonus of being excellent for the environment: their roots fix nitrogen in the soil, reducing the need for petroleum-based fertilizers.

The term *legumes* usually refer to pulses—the edible plant seeds that are harvested dry for consumption. In other words, these are the dry beans and lentils you can find in the bulk bins of any natural food store.

4. **Beets**: The pigment that makes beets purple, called betalin, is a very powerful anti-inflammatory.

5. **Bell Peppers**: Red peppers in particular contain vitamin C and antioxidants, including beta-carotene, quercetin, and luteolin.

6. **Berries**: Blueberries, raspberries, blackberries, and strawberries contain flavonoid antioxidants and anthocyanins, which turn off the inflammatory response in the body. Blueberries also have quercetin, an antioxidant that has a strong anti-inflammatory effect. The resveratrol found in berries destroys free radicals. Vitamin C is present supporting the immune system and fighting inflammation.

7. **Black Pepper**: Contains piperine, which fights acute inflammation. Piperine can increase the potency of other anti-inflammatory foods.

8. **Broccoli and Other Cruciferous Vegetables**: Cauliflower, Brussels sprouts, cabbage, and kale are also cruciferous vegetables. They are a source of sulforaphane, an anti-inflammatory antioxidant. They are high in vitamin K, which helps to regulate the inflammatory response. The potassium and magnesium they contain serve to flush out toxins. Inflammation-fighting flavonoids and carotenoids are also found in cruciferous vegetables. This family of vegetables is a superfood.

9. **Carrots**: Contain beta-carotene, which can be converted to vitamin A. On its own, it is a strong antioxidant.

10. **Cayenne**: The heat comes from capsaicinoids, which fight inflammation.

11. **Cherries**: Tart and sweet cherries contain anthocyanins and catechins, which turn off the inflammatory response. The vitamin C found in cherries supports a healthy immune system and fights inflammation. Cherries reduce markers of chronic inflammation, and the antioxidants can have a lasting effect.

12. **Chili Peppers**: Contain sinapic acid and ferulic acid, which reduce inflammation and oxidative stress. Hot chili peppers contain capsaicinoids, the source of their heat, which fight inflammation as well.

13. **Chia Seeds**: Chia seeds deliver antioxidant vitamins A, B, D, and E and phenolic acid. The mineral magnesium is also present to flush out toxins.

14. **Cinnamon**: Cinnamaldehyde is the flavonoid that gives cinnamon its flavor and smell. It can prevent and reduce inflammation.

15. **Dark Chocolate**: Chocolate that is at least 70 percent cacao is packed with flavanols and polyphenols, inflammation-reducing antioxidants. It contains zinc, magnesium, and iron, all of which have anti-inflammatory benefits.

16. **Extra Virgin Olive Oil**: EVOO has monounsaturated fatty acids that can reduce inflammation. Quercetin, a flavonoid/antioxidant, also fights inflammation. The fats make nutrients, vitamins, and anti-inflammatory compounds more available to the body.

17. **Extra Virgin Coconut Oil**: Coconut oil has high levels of antioxidants to fight free radicals and inflammation. It can withstand higher heat than olive oil.

18. **Flax Seeds**: A great source of fiber and polyphenols, which support the growth of anti-inflammatory bacteria in the gut.

Flax seeds are the richest source of lignans, a phytochemical that contains soluble fiber and acts as an antioxidant. Flax seeds must be ground to be digestible.

19. **Ginger**: Contains anti-inflammatory antioxidants called gingerols, which help to clear toxins from the body, boost the immune system, and regulate the inflammatory response. Ginger makes a delicious tea.

20. **Grapes**: Grapes contain a mix of antioxidants, including flavonoids and resveratrol. Red and black grapes contain anthocyanins, which turn off the inflammatory response.

21. **Oily Fish**: The best fish and shellfish to fight inflammation are wild-caught salmon, sardines, anchovies, herring, mackerel, sablefish, halibut, bluefin tuna, trout, bluefish, blue crab, oysters, bass, canned-in-water white tuna, shrimp, and caviar/roe.

    Oily fish are high in omega-3s. This fatty acid is only found in animal sources. Omega-3s reduce inflammation in the body. EPA and DHA, which are types of long-chain omega-3s, are among the most potent anti-inflammatory nutrients.

    If available, opt for wild fish. Farmed fish have a higher concentration of Omega-6s, which can be inflammatory.

22. **Onions and Other Allium Vegetables**: Garlic, red and yellow onions, scallions, shallots, chives, and leeks contain allicin, a compound that has an anti-inflammatory effect by stimulating anti-inflammatory proteins and suppressing markers of chronic inflammation.

23. **Oranges**: The abundant vitamin C in oranges acts as an antioxidant that reduces inflammation. The flavonoids in oranges, hesperidin and naringenin, also fight inflammation. The carotenoids inhibit the production of inflammation.

24. **Pineapple**: The vitamin C in pineapples helps to keep inflammation low. Bromelain, the digestive enzyme in pineapple, has anti-inflammatory and pain-relieving properties.

25. **Red Wine**: In moderation, red wine is an inflammation fighter. Like red grapes, it contains anthocyanidins, which reduce oxidative stress. It has also been shown to regulate blood sugar.

26. **Spinach and Other Dark Leafy Greens**: Arugula, bok choy, collard greens, dandelion greens, kale, mustard greens, broccoli raab, and Swiss chard are all considered dark leafy greens. They are packed with inflammation-fighting antioxidants, including vitamins A, C, and K and flavonoids as well. Dark leafy greens have a higher concentration of nutrients and phytochemicals than vegetables with lighter leaves. Spinach contains quercetin and kaempferol, flavonoids with an anti-inflammatory effect. Spinach, Swiss chard, and kale also contain carotenoids and tocopherols, which are found in vitamin E.

27. **Sweet Potatoes**: A good source of vitamins C and K, potassium, and B complex vitamins, which makes them a powerful antioxidant.

28. **Tea**: Green tea, some black teas, and matcha powder have an anti-inflammatory effect. Leaves from tea plants contain catechins, antioxidants that reduce inflammation. EGCG, which is only found in green teas, is the most powerful of all the catechins. Though black tea also has anti-inflammatory effects, green is more active.

29. **Tomatoes**: An excellent source of vitamin C, an antioxidant and anti-inflammatory. Tomatoes contain potassium, which flushes toxins from the body. Especially when cooked, tomatoes are rich in lycopene, which fights inflammation that can cause depression. Studies have shown that lycopene reduces inflammatory markers in the body. Lycopene exists in tomato skin and is in higher density in cherry tomatoes.

30. **Turmeric**: A powerful antioxidant and anti-inflammatory that contains curcumin, which is responsible for the spice's intense yellow color. It is one of the ingredients in curry powder.

SNACKS TO DOUSE INFLAMMATION

Crunchy, salty, sweet treats between meals might be tempting, but your efforts to get control of inflammation include paying attention to what you eat when you snack. To get you going, I have some suggestions for delicious, pain-relieving snacks. Be creative. There are so many possible combinations you can experiment with:

- Guacamole with crudités: raw carrot, pepper, broccoli, cauliflower, jicama, or any raw vegetable

- Almond butter on a celery stalk or apple slice

- Air-popped popcorn seasoned with anti-inflammatory spices and herbs, including turmeric, paprika, chili powder, fresh chopped basil, chives, rosemary, oregano

- Frozen grapes

- A handful of nuts—almonds, hazelnuts, peanuts, pecans, pistachios, and walnuts

- Hummus with crudités

- Cherry tomatoes roasted in olive oil

- Hard-boiled eggs

- Full-fat yogurt with berries, chia seeds, nuts

- Smoked salmon on whole wheat bread or crackers

- Kale chips

- Frozen melon balls

- Roasted, herbed chickpeas

- Black bean dip with crudités

- Avocado toast on whole wheat bread

- Fruit or vegetable smoothie made with yogurt

- Olives

- A couple squares of dark chocolate

- Fruit salad
- Roasted cauliflower with turmeric
- Berry freezer pops

All it takes is a bit of planning to have food on hand that will suppress inflammation. As your pain begins to subside, you will enjoy these wholesome snacks even more.

VITAMINS AND SUPPLEMENTS FOR A HEALTHY BACK

To reduce back problems, certain vitamins and nutrients are essential for nourishing the bones, muscles, discs, and other structures of the spine. Some of the nutrients act as antioxidants, which help to reduce inflammation. Though you could take supplements, I recommend getting these vitamins from natural sources. This partial list highlights some nutrients that can help to relieve back problems and pain along with a list of food sources:

Calcium

Consuming enough calcium is essential for maintaining bone mass throughout your life. Adequate calcium intake helps to prevent osteoporosis. Calcium must be balanced with vitamin D to produce strong bones.

Sources: milk, yogurt, cheese, dark green leafy vegetables, legumes, oranges, tofu, blackstrap molasses, fish rich in omega-3s.

Vitamin D3

This vitamin helps the body to absorb calcium. Low levels of vitamin D have been linked to inflammatory diseases, including rheumatoid arthritis. In the lab, vitamin D shows a significant anti-inflammatory effect on cells and can lessen the pain of chronic inflammation. Your body makes vitamin D when your skin is in sunlight, but it is found naturally in only a few foods.

Sources: fatty fish (salmon), liver, cod liver oil, beef, egg yolks. Some cereals, milk, juices, and breads are fortified with vitamin D.

Magnesium

Magnesium is a mineral that helps to keep bones strong. By maintaining bone density, this mineral helps to prevent back problems. It takes part in more than 300 biochemical reactions in the body. If levels of magnesium drop in the blood, the body pulls magnesium from the bones, which is not a good thing for your spine. Magnesium helps to relax and contract muscles and strengthens the muscles that support the spine.

Sources: green leafy vegetables, fish, beans, seeds, nuts, whole grains, yogurt, avocados, bananas, and 70 percent cacao dark chocolate.

Vitamin C

This antioxidant helps to eliminate free radicals, which can trigger inflammation by damaging cells and tissue. As an antioxidant, vitamin C helps to heal injured muscles, tendons, ligaments, and intervertebral discs, and keeps the vertebrae strong.

Vitamin C is necessary for the production of collagen found in bones, muscles, skin, and tendons. Collagen is part of the tissue-forming process.

Vitamin C is also believed to lower levels of C-reactive protein (CRP), which is made by the liver. CRP is a marker of inflammation. One theory is that vitamin C may be suppressing the production of cytokines, which regulate the inflammatory process. When cytokines are suppressed, inflammation is reduced.

Sources: citrus fruits, strawberries, peppers, broccoli, Brussels sprouts, spinach, leafy greens, berries, and sweet potatoes.

Vitamin B12

B12 contributes to the formation of bone-building cells and is necessary for the formation of red blood cells in the bone marrow. Vitamin B complex is believed to help nerve pain.

Sources: animal proteins, such as eggs, fish, poultry, and meat, and dairy products including milk, yogurt, and cheese. Because B12 is not found in vegetables, vegetarians should consider taking supplements.

Vitamin K2

K2 directs bone minerals by distributing calcium from the soft tissues and depositing the calcium into the bones. The combination of K2 and calcium works to keep bones in the spine and throughout the body strong and healthy. K1 is the plant form of K2.

Sources K2: healthy fats of meats, cheeses, egg yolks, and other dairy products. Sources K1: green leafy vegetables like spinach and kale and broccoli.

Iron

Iron plays a role in the conversion of vitamin D to its active form. It is also involved in the production of collagen. Iron is a component of hemoglobin and myoglobin, proteins that deliver oxygen throughout the body, including tissues that support the spine.

Sources: liver, pork, fish, shellfish, red meat, poultry, green leafy vegetables, lentils, beans, eggs, soy, and whole grains.

Glucosamine and Chondroitin

Glucosamine, an amino acid, is found in high concentrations in cartilage and connective tissue. Chondroitin is found in connective tissues and is often taken with glucosamine. Glucosamine and chondroitin are structural components of cartilage, the tissue that cushions the joints. Both are produced naturally in the body. They are also available as dietary supplements. Researchers have studied the effects of these supplements, individually or in combination, on osteoarthritis, which destroys cartilage in the joints. They are known to relieve joint pain due to inflammation.

If you want to watch your back, changing your eating habits can advance the progress you have already made with more and better movement. Adopting the diet outlined in this chapter will supercharge your energy, lift your spirits, and heal your pain.

Chapter 10

Strategy 7:
A Good Night's Sleep

More than half of people with back pain report significant sleep problems. Chronic pain makes it difficult for many to fall asleep, and that pain can interrupt sleep. Simply changing position while sleeping can trigger pain. A vicious cycle is set in motion. Chronic pain disrupts restful sleep, making you more tired and consequently more sensitive to pain the next day. In turn, your intensified experience of pain makes sleeping more difficult. Sleep and pain appear to be reciprocally related, but studies show that poor sleep may have a stronger influence on the experience of chronic pain. What is certain is that chronic pain and sleep problems are an unhealthy combination.

Restorative sleep is vital for optimal physical, mental, and emotional health. While you sleep, your brain repairs and regenerates cells, tissue, and nerves, boosting your hormone and immune systems. Healthy sleep is divided into four stages. As you progress through the first two stages you become increasingly unplugged from the world. In the third stage, you reach deep, restorative sleep, when your brain and body activity drop to their lowest point during the sleep cycle. Deep sleep is crucial for physical renewal, hormonal regulation, and growth. The fourth stage is REM (rapid eye movement) sleep. During this stage, your brain processes and synthesizes memories and emotions, which are directly connected to learning and higher-level thinking.

A good night's sleep is made up of several rounds of the four stages of the sleep cycle. In a typical night, a person goes through three to six sleep cycles.

Each cycle lasts about ninety minutes. If you do not sleep long enough to complete several cycles, you are not getting enough deep and REM sleep. Not getting enough restorative sleep has profound consequences that affect your thinking, emotions, and physical health. Sleepers who wake frequently during the first two stages may have difficulty cycling into the deeper sleep stages. People with insomnia may not get enough total sleep to accumulate the needed time in each stage. The importance of getting a good night's sleep cannot be underestimated.

You have probably noticed that after a full night's sleep you think clearly and feel at your best physically. But did you know that getting between seven and nine hours of sleep a night also improves your body's ability to keep inflammation in check at a cellular level? Not getting adequate sleep is likely to make you more vulnerable to the physical and emotional effects of stress. A chronic sleep-stress cycle is a trigger for inflammation. Sleeping well provides protection against stress and works to keep inflammation in check. As a result, one of the key effects of a good night's sleep is a reduction in chronic pain.

A PAIN IN THE NECK

While I was writing orders after surgery, an anesthesiologist asked me if I had a moment to talk. I invited her to have a seat.

Looking up from my papers, I asked, "What's up?"

"I have a chronic, nagging pain in my neck that radiates to my shoulders. I've been unable to sleep more than four hours a night. My family is suffering because I am overtired and stressed out. I'm depressed and anxious and don't know what to do. I manage to do my work, but personally, I am a mess."

I sent her for an MRI scan of her cervical spine, which showed mild degeneration at C5-C6. When we met to discuss what the scan revealed, I noticed her poor posture. She was slouching, and her head jutted forward as she moved. Her poor posture was clearly contributing to her pain. I advised her about the importance of maintaining proper posture: a neutral spine with her ears over her shoulders and her shoulder blades pulled back and drawn together. I told her about a study done at San Francisco State University, which found a link between poor posture and depression. I explained that many experts believe stooping and slouching to be associated with weight gain, heart burn, anxiety, and respiratory conditions.

I began by introducing her to several posture correcting exercises. I taught her how to practice deep belly breathing to open up her chest. Deep belly breathing technique enables the spinal nerves to move within the spinal channels, diminishing pain. I showed her a series of back and neck stretches to ease the tension and increase her range of motion. I recommended that she add more movement in her life and take long, hot showers.

When we discussed her insomnia, she told me that she usually watched TV in bed while she was trying to go to sleep. I explained that the blue light of the television screen could be stimulating her, which would make it more difficult for her to fall asleep. While we discussed her busy schedule, I realized she often skipped lunch and had a big dinner at 8 p.m. with a glass or two of wine. Going to bed on a full stomach was not going to contribute to a night's restful sleep. Drinking alcohol close to the time you go to bed may help you fall asleep but can disrupt sleep later. Alcohol has been shown to reduce sleep quality and duration. In addition, the wine she had with dinner could cause her to get up to use the bathroom during the night. We reviewed what we could do to change her bedtime routine to relax her and induce sleep.

"I'm so tired of being tired, I'll try anything," she said. She resolved to overhaul her sleeping habits.

After two weeks, she was able to get a good night's sleep. She reported that she was a new person and had her happy life back. Adopting some of the strategies of the Watch Your Back program had brought back her sense of well-being, and her neck pain disappeared.

YOUR INTERNAL CLOCK
AND INFLAMMATION

Your body has an internal clock with a daily biological rhythm, called a circadian rhythm, which regulates your active and rest states with biochemical reactions synchronized to light and dark. Your internal clock regulates physical, mental, and behavioral changes that follow a daily cycle. Your circadian rhythms drive the production of hormones and other physiological changes that move you between sleep and wakefulness during a twenty-four-hour day. Just as your sleep-wake cycle is controlled by your body's internal clock, many other bodily functions wax and wane in response to the twenty-four-hour circadian rhythm. For example, normal body temperature is lowest at about 5 a.m., when it averages 97°F, and highest at about 5 p.m., when it averages 99.4°F. Hormone levels fluctuate as well. Cortisol secretion is most elevated during the morning to get you going. Melatonin, the "dark hormone," is produced by the brain's pineal gland at night to make you tired. In a sense, your circadian rhythm keeps you on schedule.

That same rhythm regulates your immune system, which controls the level of inflammation in your body. Let me repeat that important point: sleep and inflammation are regulated by the same biorhythms. When poor sleep disrupts your circadian rhythms, your immune system goes haywire, resulting in inflammation and pain. Getting good sleep is essential because sleep, immune function, and inflammation share a common regulator. Too little sleep raises levels of inflammation in your body. Just one night of insufficient sleep is enough to activate inflammation throughout the body. Consistently getting the right amount of sleep—between seven and nine hours for most adults—helps to avoid systemic, low-grade inflammation. A full night of restful sleep makes a difference at a cellular level in your body's ability to keep inflammation in check.

GET IN SYNC WITH YOUR CIRCADIAN RHYTHMS

You need a consistent sleep routine to coordinate your sleep and immune system, which governs inflammation. One simple way to accomplish this is to go to bed and get up at the same time every day.

ARE YOU AN EARLY BIRD OR A NIGHT OWL?

In considering how to get good sleep, you have to be aware of your chronotype, which is when you are genetically disposed to sleep. Are you an early bird or a night owl, in other words, a morning person or a night person? If you sleep when your chronotype dictates it, you will get higher-quality sleep. I consider following your chronotype to be so important that there are two Watch Your Back programs: one for early birds and one for night owls.

Your chronotype is genetic, determined by the genes that regulate your inner clock. Your chronotype can be manipulated to a degree by light exposure, light timing, exercise schedules, social interactions, and sleep schedules. If you are an early bird, set an appropriate bedtime and stick with it. If you wake up early, do a morning workout. Exercising later in the day or in the evening can make it harder to go to sleep for early birds. Night owls should arrange their schedules so that their days start later. There are several things you can do to follow your circadian rhythm:

- Do not expose yourself to bright lights, specifically blue light, within one or two hours of bedtime. Your brain sets its circadian rhythm by its exposure to light. If you watch TV, play games on your smart phone, or read on your tablet, the blue light of those electronic devices makes your brain think that it is light out and that you need to be awake.

- Enjoy sunlight in the morning after you wake up. Exercising outside is ideal exposure. Your brain will wake your body up.

- Temperature influences your inner clock. Exercising in the morning raises your temperature, a wake-up call for your brain. Reducing the temperature of your room at night will send a sleep signal to your brain.

- Make sure your bedroom is dark. Do not use bathroom light when you are getting ready for bed. A night light or a dimmer will expose you to a minimal amount of light. Some people wear a sleep mask while they sleep to block out any light.

- Follow your chronotype when you choose a regular bedtime.

HOW TO GET A GOOD NIGHT'S SLEEP WITH CHRONIC PAIN

Insomnia is a term that refers to several sleep problems, namely difficulty falling asleep, difficulty staying asleep, and waking up earlier than intended. Many of my patients suffering from chronic back pain do not feel refreshed in the morning. Their sleep is not restorative. They are not getting the deep sleep they need. Many have several changes in their sleep state every hour that pull them out of deep, restorative sleep. The quality of their sleep is light and fails to refresh them. Non-restorative sleep results in low energy, depressed mood, and more intense pain.

When it comes to going to sleep, people with chronic pain need a different set of guidelines. The standard recommendation for those who have trouble relaxing and falling asleep is to eliminate distractions by turning off lights and making it quiet. Creating such a quiet environment can cause problems for people with chronic pain. Lying in bed trying to fall asleep only makes them focus more on the pain. One of the most effective pain management methods is distraction. During the day, you can keep busy and engage in activities that keep your mind off your pain, but trying to fall asleep can bring your awareness of the pain front and center. The next two chapters will reveal ways to use your mind to divert your attention from your pain. What follows is a list of tips on how to get a good night's sleep:

- Exercise regularly, but not within a few hours of bedtime. People who exercise regularly sleep better at night. They fall asleep faster, and they sleep longer than sedentary people. The more vigorously you exercise, the more you benefit. Not only does exercise tire you out, but it also relieves stress, which is what is keeping you awake.

- Go to bed and wake up at the same time every day, including weekends. Observing a schedule will train your body to sleep.

- Skip naps during the day if naps make sleeping at night more difficult. When you do nap, restrict your naps to fifteen to twenty minutes in the early afternoon.

- Wind down late in the day. If you can, schedule stressful or demanding activities in the morning and less challenging things to do later.

- Avoid eating heavy meals at night.

- Avoid caffeine late in the day. You should stop drinking coffee by mid-afternoon. Caffeine can keep you awake up to twelve hours after drinking it.

- Do not smoke, especially near bedtime or if you wake up in the night.

- Avoid drinking alcohol after dinner. You may fall asleep faster when you drink, but the quality of your sleep suffers. Alcohol causes wakefulness in the second half of the night.

- Avoid sugar, which you are already doing, but it is especially important at night. It is too stimulating and raises inflammation levels.

- Loosen your back muscles before bedtime. Do some gentle stretches to help release muscle tension.

- Have a relaxing bedtime routine and do the same thing every night before going to sleep. You could read, take a bath with scented bath salts, have a cup of warm milk or chamomile tea, meditate, or listen to soothing music. Your mind will connect these activities with sleep.

- Use your bedroom only for sleeping or having sex. Do not watch TV or talk on the phone in bed.

- Turn off or at least mute your cell phone.

- Do not lie in bed worrying about things. Set aside another time, maybe after dinner, to think about what you can do about what is bothering you. If you are overloaded, get out of bed and make a list, then think of something pleasant.

- Have a relaxed attitude about sleep. Do not obsess about not being able to fall asleep, it will only make you anxious and frustrated. If you have a sleepless night, do not let it throw you. Just go with it. Console yourself by assuming the next night will be better.

- Try belly breathing or other relaxation techniques, which you will learn about in chapter 12, to reduce your perception of pain and take your mind off your inability to sleep.

- If you cannot sleep after about twenty minutes, get up and go to another room. Sit quietly for about twenty minutes before going back to bed.

- If all else fails, turn to sleeping medication. This should be a last resort. You do not want relying on sleep medications to become a habit. Always consult with a doctor about taking any sleeping aids like Benadryl or melatonin. Take prescribed medications with great caution.

BEST SLEEPING POSITIONS

The best sleeping position is one that gives you the best rest. You might sleep in different positions during the night. To reduce back pain using extra pillows for support can help. The soreness you might feel when you get up in the morning may not result from your sleeping position alone.

Pain at the end of the day or in the morning can be the residual effect of bad posture or movement that is responsible for the pain in the first place.

As I have mentioned before, movement and gravity can compress your discs, like a sponge being squeezed. While you are lying down, your discs fill with fluid. They are plump with fluid in the morning. As you start to move against gravity once you are out of bed, your plumped-up discs can make you more sensitive to back pain.

Your sleeping position can put added stress on your neck, back, and hips. Some commentary on the four most common sleeping positions will help you to eliminate potential problems.

Side Sleeping: The Most Popular Position

Though side sleeping is the most common position, sleeping on your side can lead to neck, shoulder, and hip pain. Side sleeping can lead to jaw tightness on the side on which you are lying. Another negative: sleeping on your side can contribute to facial wrinkles. You might be interested to know that one study found that sleeping on your left side can reduce snoring and is good for digestion, while sleeping on your right side can increase heartburn and acid reflux.

In finding a good sleeping position, your goal is to keep your spine in a neutral position, close to a straight line, parallel with the surface of the bed. With a neutral spine, muscle and joint tension is minimal, and the curves of your spine are maintained.

The angle of your neck is important. If your pillow is too thin or too thick, your neck will curve up or down, which can strain your neck muscles. The entire length of your neck needs to be supported, otherwise it will be out of alignment. Traditional pillows support your head rather than your neck. Cervical or contoured pillows do a better job of keeping your neck and head aligned with your spine.

The position of your hips can have a dramatic impact on the quality of your sleep. When you are lying on your side, your hips should be perpendicular to the bed. The side of your hip that is touching the bed should be directly below the opposite side. Keeping your hips aligned with each other helps to prevent twisting the spine, which increases tension.

Slightly lift your knees up toward your chest to reduce pressure on your back.

Many side sleepers use a pillow between their knees, especially if they have lower back pain. Doing so helps to support a neutral position of the hips. Specialty knee pillows are available.

Side sleeping requires a balance of support and give in your mattress. If your mattress is too firm and the weight of your body is carried by your shoulders and hips, your spine is forced to curve differently. The same thing can happen if your mattress is too soft.

Back Sleeping: Considered the Best Sleeping Position for a Healthy Back

Sleeping on your back offers the most health benefits. This position evenly distributes weight to the full length of the body's largest surface. Back sleeping minimizes pressure points and ensures good alignment of the head, neck, and spine. Many find that putting a small pillow under the knees provides additional support and helps to maintain the spine's natural curve. A pillow under your knees can help to flatten your back and open up the spaces where irritated nerves might be compressed.

When you lie flat on your back, your head should be facing the ceiling. Avoid twisting your head to either side to avoid straining your neck. Use a pillow to support your head and neck, one under your knees, and fill in any gaps between your body and the mattress—under your lower back, for example.

Stomach Sleeping

Sleeping on your stomach is not ideal if you have neck pain, but it can be a good position if your pain is in your lower back. Lying on your stomach puts your low back in a more extended position with an arch in your spine. If you become uncomfortable, place a pillow underneath your hips and waist to raise your mid-section, which will help to improve spinal alignment. The pillow opens up space for the nerves in your low back to decompress and reduces tension. Consider using a flat pillow under your head or sleep without one.

Stomach sleeping is considered not to be the best for posture because the head is usually turned to one side, which can twist the spine and puts additional stress on the neck and shoulders. If you lie face down, using a small, firm pillow or a tightly rolled-up towel can prop up your forehead and give you breathing space.

Fetal Position

If you have a herniated disc, a curled-up position can relieve the pain. This position is good for your lower back and works well during pregnancy. An added benefit is that it reduces snoring. Lying on your side with your knees tucked into your chest helps to open up the spinal joints.

Your posture should be loose and relaxed and your back relatively straight. If you curl up too tightly, you could limit your breathing. If you have issues with joint pain or stiffness, sleeping in a tight fetal position might make you sore when you get up in the morning. Use a pillow to support your head and neck. A pillow between your knees could make the position more comfortable.

Sleeping While Pregnant

Side sleeping is generally recommended during pregnancy, especially in late pregnancy, to avoid compression of the blood flow to the uterus. Sleeping on the left side allows for optimal blood flow and takes the pressure off the kidneys and liver, which helps with swelling in the hands, ankles, and feet.

Stomach sleeping can work until weeks sixteen to eighteen. At that point, the belly has gotten big enough and breasts tender enough to make sleeping on the stomach uncomfortable. Some women use a donut-shaped pillow to accommodate their growing belly.

Sleeping on the back is considered safe during the first trimester. Back sleeping can cause problems with backaches, breathing, the digestive system, and hemorrhoids. More important, back sleeping can cause a decrease in circulation to the baby. Using a wedge pillow will allow blood flow to the fetus.

Best Postures for Reading or Watching TV in Bed

People love to lie down while reading or watching TV. After a busy day, there is nothing like collapsing on a comfortable couch or welcoming bed to unwind. Taking care of your back even when you are relaxing will help you to stay pain free.

Sitting upright in bed, when properly supported, seems to keep people comfortable for a long read or binge watching. You should place your back straight against the headboard or use a reading pillow with arms to support your back. This prevents neck and back pain and helps you read comfortably for hours. You should hold your book or electronic device about a foot away from you. You will have to hold up what you are reading to avoid tilting your head too much to avoid text neck.

When you lie down to read or view, the force exerted by the body is transmitted to the object you are lying on that supports you. Though gravity is eliminated, you still need to be careful that your spine is aligned properly: neck aligned above the shoulder, back aligned above the buttocks for equal balance transfer of spine forces.

The supine position is the most popular. Be sure your back stays straight. The main challenge when you read on your back is to hold your book or screen appropriately to avoid eye strain. Hold the book above your face to protect your neck and back from getting strained. Some people use prism glasses to avoid eyestrain or tired arms. If you tend to sink into your bed, back and neck pain can develop. You can use a pillow from your shoulder blades to the lumbar region to keep your back aligned.

Reading while lying on your side is another popular position. It allows for flexibility because you can fold your legs at the knees or keep them stretched out. It is a good idea to bend your top leg slightly so that your calf is supported. This position ensures proper blood circulation. It's easier to hold a book when you lie on your side, but your hands may get tired if you stay in this position for a long time. Be sure to put your head on a firm pillow to keep your shoulders and head slightly elevated. If you are right-handed, it is advisable to lie on your right side and hold the book in your right hand. The reverse holds true if you are left-handed.

I do not recommend reading or watching television in a prone position. This position can force you to extend your neck, hike your shoulders to your ears, place your wrists and elbows in awkward positions, and jar your pelvis. Reading on your stomach can promote pain in the lumbar region because your spine remains arched. The muscles in your neck and shoulders are tense when you prop yourself up. If you want to read or view in this position, put a roller cushion under your breast, support your chin on a pillow, and read or watch without being too close to the book or screen. Do not alter the curvature of your neck.

If you are binge-watching TV, it's a good idea to get up and move around at least once an hour. You can do stretches during commercials or your active breaks.

SLEEP EQUIPMENT

Your mattress, pillows, bedding, and other sleep accessories can create a sleep-inducing environment. If you have difficulty sleeping, you should see what changes you can make to your bedroom that will help you to fall asleep and stay asleep.

On Mattresses

A good mattress is a must if you suffer from chronic pain. Though firm mattresses are often recommended, medium firm may work better for people with chronic lower back pain. Body shape, size, and proportions can determine how much support you need. Wide hips may be better suited to a softer mattress, while slim hips might require a firmer one to keep the spine properly aligned. Though softer mattresses can seem more comfortable, they provide less support. Sinking too deep can throw the spine out of natural alignment. In general, back sleepers need a firmer mattress and side sleepers a softer one. Because most people change positions during the night, a medium-firm mattress is the best bet. There are several ways to adjust the firmness of your mattress. You can use a foam mattress topper to add additional support or put a plywood board underneath the mattress to increase firmness. Or you could invest in a smart mattress that adjusts to your different positions as you sleep.

Whether your mattress heats you up is another issue to consider. Foam mattresses, in particular, can compress and trap your body heat after a few hours, which may make you warmer and disturb your sleep. Many of my patients complain of waking up in a sweat. Cooling mattress toppers and cooling blankets are available to solve that problem.

If you are buying a new mattress, make sure to try out many to find one that works for you. You spend a lot of time on top of your mattress. It is worth taking the time to find one that helps you sleep. You should get a new mattress every ten years.

On Pillows

A pillow for your head should maintain the natural posture of your neck and help to support the spine. It should be adaptable to different positions:

- If you sleep primarily on your back, a thin pillow will work better for you. If your head is raised too much, you will be putting additional strain on your neck and back. Memory foam can be a good choice because it is firm and molds to the shape of your head and neck.

- If you sleep on your side, a thicker pillow may be a better choice. For optimal support, the pillow should completely fill the space between your neck and the mattress. A gusseted pillow is a good choice for side sleepers.

- Stomach sleepers should use a thin pillow or no pillow at all. Pushing your head up and back can put pressure on your neck. A small pillow that only props up your forehead is an option.

You should replace your pillows every twelve to eighteen months to guarantee adequate support.

Special Pillows

Special orthopedic pillows can offer extra support for your neck. Called cervical pillows, they fill the spaces under the head and neck. This type of pillow has a deeper depression where the head lies and offers extra support under the neck.

Rather than using separate pillows for your head and knees, a body pillow the length of your entire body works well if you sleep on your side. The top of the pillow can support your head and neck and the bottom your knees and legs. Body pillows work well for pregnant women because they provide extra support for the abdomen.

Wedge pillows recreate the recliner position in bed, which is good for chronic back pain.

Sleep Accessories

There are countless gadgets and products designed to reduce distractions, make you comfortable, calm you, and improve your ability to fall asleep and get restorative sleep. Doing a search for what is available is eye-opening because so much is out there. It becomes clear that the market for things that promote sleep is substantial. Leaving out teddy bears, I am listing just a few items my patients have mentioned:

- Masks, from cool and silky to weighted
- Earplugs
- White noise machines
- Blackout blinds and curtains
- Cooling sheets
- Memory foam pillows
- Weighted blankets
- Air purifiers/fans
- Calming essential oil infusers
- Dimming alarm clocks

Using any of these props or others you find appealing can become part of your bedtime ritual.

15 FOODS THAT PROMOTE SLEEPINESS

Some foods can help you get better sleep, mainly because they contain nutrients believed to reduce anxiety and make you sleepy. You will recognize some from the "30 Inflammation Extinguishers" listed in the preceding chapter. The list identifies ingredients that make each food sleep promoting:

1. Almonds: magnesium

2. Bananas: magnesium, potassium, and tryptophan

3. Chamomile tea: apigenin, an antioxidant that promotes sleepiness

4. Cherries: high levels of melatonin

5. Fatty fish: vitamin D and omega-3 fatty acids increase the production of serotonin

6. Honey: glucose in honey reduces the level of orexin in the brain, which makes you alert

7. Kiwi: serotonin, antioxidants, vitamin C, and carotenoids

8. Milk: tryptophan

9. Oatmeal: melatonin and complex carbs

10. Passionflower tea: apigenin, an antioxidant that reduces anxiety and promotes sleepiness

11. Pumpkin seeds: tryptophan

12. Sweet potatoes: complex carbohydrates and potassium

13. Turkey: tryptophan

14. Walnuts: magnesium, melatonin, omega-3 fatty acids

15. Yogurt: melatonin

If you want a snack between dinner and bedtime any of these foods would be a good choice. Anything that improves the quality of your sleep is an effective weapon against inflammation.

THE JOYS OF POWER NAPPING

Just one night of bad sleep takes a toll on your body. When you lose sleep one night, you feel it the next day. Sleep is cumulative. If chronic back pain interferes with your sleep several days in a row, you build up a sleep deficit. Such a deficit affects you in several ways, including reaction time, judgment, motivation, short-term memory, and patience. You can recover, relax, and recharge with a "power nap." Naps are an effective way to make up that sleep deficit.

If you are concerned that napping might make it harder to fall asleep at night, power napping may be the answer. The idea is to nap no longer than fifteen to twenty minutes. Napping too long can make you wake up groggy. You will wake up refreshed from a "cat nap." A short nap can boost your energy and mood and make you more alert.

Do not nap late in the day, which is more likely to disturb your sleep. If you are an early bird, the best time to nap is 1–1:30 p.m. If you are a night owl, your optimal naptime is 2:30–3 p.m. Think of the wisdom of cultures that build a siesta into the day. They knew what they were doing.

It may seem counter-intuitive, but some say that gulping down a cup of coffee just before power napping can enhance your productivity. Coffee takes time to start showing its effects, usually around twenty minutes, the ideal length of time for your nap. By the time the caffeine kicks in, you will wake up with double the energy. The nap combined with the stimulating effect of coffee will energize you.

If the caffeine approach is not for you, set an alarm to make sure you do not oversleep. If you want to take a fifteen- to twenty-minute nap, it might take you five minutes to fall asleep. With that in mind, set your alarm for twenty to twenty-five minutes.

Finding a place to nap is easy if you are working from home. Choose any comfortable spot, but be sure it is not too comfortable, otherwise you might want to extend your nap and avoid getting back to the demands of the day. Many corporations now recognize the importance of power naps, so they have introduced nap pods or nap rooms in their offices. Employees can take a short nap and resume work with increased efficiency. If your office doesn't have a dedicated space for a nap, consider napping in your car, your office, or your cubby.

The next chapter focuses on the psychological aspect of the program. Is your cup half full or half empty? Your answer to that question has a lot to do with how you manage chronic pain.

Chapter 11

Strategy 8:
Choose to Be Positive

Having a positive mental attitude can help you to keep back pain in context and overcome it. The experience of pain is subjective. Changing the way you think about your chronic pain can affect how your body responds to it. You may not be able to stop the physical pain, but you can control how your mind handles the pain. The way you think about your situation influences how you feel and what you do. In other words, if your thoughts about your pain are negative and revolve around being helpless, you will feel pain more intensely than you would if you approach your condition in a hopeful and constructive way.

These observations brilliantly capture the difference between a positive or negative take on life:

"We can complain because rose bushes have thorns
or rejoice because thorn bushes have roses."
—Abraham Lincoln

"The optimist sees the donut; the pessimist sees the hole."
—Oscar Wilde

"A pessimist sees the difficulty in every opportunity; an
optimist sees the opportunity in every difficulty."
—Winston Churchill

"Choose to be optimistic. It feels better."
—Dalai Lama

Being negative disrupts how you interact with your environment by affecting your ability to perceive and remember. Negativity slows down the creation of new neural connections. Being positive improves your ability to be more alert and productive because an upbeat outlook stimulates the growth of nerve connections, increasing mental productivity and the ability to analyze and think. Another significant benefit is that positive thinking stimulates the production of serotonin, the "feel-good" neurotransmitter, a chemical messenger in the brain that stabilizes mood, feelings of well-being, and happiness.

Researchers have found that being optimistic can improve your overall health. Choosing to have a positive outlook can boost your immune system and counter depression. Even more important, positivity is an effective tool for stress management. As you have learned, stress can lead to low-grade inflammation, which intensifies pain. When your responses are optimistic, you are better able to handle everyday stress, which will reduce your back pain both physically and psychologically.

Nerve tracts—carrying pain signals up to the brain and down from the brain—regulate the sensitivity of the spinal cord. This communication determines how much pain you feel. When your brain thinks the pain is important, your experience will be amplified. When your brain considers the pain inconsequential, it will be reduced. Attention accounts for your experience of pain. Most chronic pain is attributed more to sensitization of the nervous system than to injuries in the parts of your body that hurt.

My aim in this chapter is to help you to identify negative thinking, change your outlook, and take constructive action, all of which will help you feel better. I want you to learn to observe the thoughts that seem to be automatic and how those thoughts affect your emotions without your realizing it. I demonstrate how to evaluate the accuracy of your automatic assumptions, which you can do only by developing the skill to notice, interrupt, and correct the negativity that routinely seeps into your thinking.

You can learn to tamp down negative thoughts and look at the bright side. That is easy enough said, but you might wonder how to replace negative thoughts with positive ones. The core of this chapter is a discussion of skills and techniques for fostering positive thoughts and emotions in your everyday life. If you shift your outlook from negative to positive, you will become more self-accepting and less critical of the world around you. When your responses are optimistic, you are better able to handle everyday stress, which will reduce your back pain both physically and psychologically.

LIVING LIFE TO THE FULLEST

Mary was full of life at 100. She loved to spend time with her four grandchildren and to work in her beautiful garden. She was a great cook and always ate well. Mary still loved to entertain and often shared wonderful meals with friends and family.

Without warning, she sustained two vertebral compression fractures. The condition is most commonly caused by osteoporosis. In the United States, close to 750,000 spinal fractures occur annually due to osteoporosis-weakened bones. Mary's back pain was so severe that she was unable to walk or stand. This vivacious woman was bed- and wheelchair-bound for four months. For a person as active as Mary, this restricted state was a radical change. She was determined to get back on her feet again.

Her medical doctor attempted brace and medication therapy. Nothing worked. Mary would not give up. She was not about to let her condition deprive her of her independence and favorite activities. Her doctor referred Mary to me.

I was very impressed when we met. She was remarkable for a woman her age. She had no medical problems, passed a full cardiac stress test, and was mentally sharp. For many of my patients in their eighties, medical problems make surgery too risky. That was not the case with Mary.

I was able to do a minimally invasive spinal procedure to stabilize the vertebral fracture and to prevent further collapse. We were able to avoid general anesthesia and provided conscious sedation anesthesia. With great care, the surgery only took twenty minutes. Six months later, Mary was no longer immobilized. She got around with a walker or a cane. Most important, she was pain free.

Mary was able to undergo surgery because she took care of herself her entire life. Her optimism and energy contributed to her resilience and good health. Genetics aside, she is a shining example of how the right attitude and proper self-care can prevent premature aging and can extend life's active and productive years.

Mary led a full life after her surgery. She passed away with her family around her when she was 105 years old.

THE SUNNY SIDE OF THE STREET

Positivity does not mean you should be happy all the time. That would be impossible. Having a positive mindset is not about being cheerful. It is more about believing in yourself and the outcomes of your efforts. Having a positive outlook is a tendency to focus on the good in your life. I am not saying that you should ignore the bad things. Having a positive attitude means that you address the challenges in your life by making the most of any situation you find yourself in and by seeing the best in people. Positivity means approaching unpleasant situations in a positive and productive way. There are several qualities, all of which you can cultivate, that are intrinsic to a positive mindset:

Optimism

An optimist believes that the outcomes of experiences will generally be positive. Optimists are willing to make an effort and take a chance instead of thinking their efforts will not be successful. Optimism is the way people explain the cause of events. Optimists tend to see failure or bad experiences as temporary rather than permanent, external rather than internal, and specific rather than broad.

Acceptance

Thinking positively will not protect you from reality. A positive person understands that things do not always work out as wanted but learns from mistakes.

Resilience

When faced with disappointment, failure, loss, adversity, or sadness, a positive person bounces back instead of folding and giving up. In extremely difficult times, a positive person does not deny or suppress the pain, sadness, or devastation but allows himself or herself to experience the pain and emotions.

Gratitude

This is an important quality. It means appreciating the good things in your life. Positive thinkers are always appreciative of something.

Mindfulness

Positive people are aware of how their minds work. They are conscious of when their minds turn on them. When negativity creeps in, they shift their focus to the upside of any situation.

Integrity

Positive people are not dishonest or self-absorbed. The ability to see the good in others helps to shape their own principled behavior.

A POSITIVITY CATALOG

You know a positive person when you see one. A positive attitude produces identifiable traits and behaviors. When you need to remind yourself to approach a situation in a positive way, a look at the following list of traits will give you cues about positively charged attitudes and behaviors.

A positive person is:

Accepting	Determined	Positive
Adaptable	Engaged	Practical
Adventurous	Enthusiastic	Pro-active
Affable	Expansive	Realistic
Agreeable	Faithful	Reliable
Ambitious	Flexible	Responsible
Amiable	Focused	Responsive
Aspiring	Forgiving	Self-confident
Brave	Friendly	Self-directed
Bright	Generous	Self-disciplined
Broad-minded	Grateful	Self-reliant
Candid	Hard-working	Selfless
Caring	Helpful	Sensitive
Cheerful	Honest	Sincere
Communicative	Inclusive	Supportive
Compassionate	Interested	Sympathetic
Conscientious	Involved	Thoughtful
Considerate	Kind	Tolerant
Cooperative	Motivated	Trusting
Courageous	Open-minded	Unpretentious
Curious	Optimistic	Unselfish
Decisive	Persevering	Willing

Imagine yourself in just about any challenging situation. You will find a word to describe the upbeat way to handle it in this list.

RECOGNIZING NEGATIVE SELF-TALK

Self-talk is the chatter that goes on all the time in your head. Often that chatter has to do with what went wrong, what is wrong, and what can go wrong. Negative self-talk can discourage and limit you. It is full of self-criticism that erodes your self-confidence and deprives you of hope. That pessimistic self-talk keeps you from recognizing or taking advantage of opportunities. In contrast, positive self-talk is encouraging and appreciative. Your inner voice can motivate you toward a goal.

Your brain naturally tends toward negativity. It looks for, learns from, and holds on to anything it considers a danger. It's about survival of the fittest. Your ancient ancestors were likely to live long enough to pass on their genes by remembering where they confronted a predator. Because of this evolutionary trait, your brain perceives negative stimuli more rapidly and easily than positive ones. Your brain is more sensitive to the negative and tends to develop negative thought patterns.

To avoid getting stuck in a negative mode of thinking, you have to become aware of the thought patterns that can be shaping your experience of the world. Problems like anxiety, depression, and self-defeating behavior can be broken down into similar thought patterns. When you experience prolonged pain, negative thinking can dominate your thoughts about your back problems. Thinking "I can't take this" or "it's never going to get better" can exacerbate your pain and inhibit your recovery. The fact is that if you tell yourself you can't do something, you begin to believe it.

In order to break out of negative thinking, you must recognize the automatic negative thought patterns that determine your response to the world. These negative ways of thinking may have become so habitual that you do not even notice them. The problem is that thinking in this way triggers high levels of stress in your body.

One of the best ways to reduce your experience of pain is to change these negative thought patterns. As I describe various negative thought patterns, you will see that they distort reality in a way that defeats you. It is in your power to transform from negativity to positivity. You can shift gears and establish new thought patterns. One way to start is to identify how your thinking may shape your automatic response to events. There are many negative thought patterns. What follows is an introduction to some of the many negative thought patterns with examples of the self-talk that accompanies each one.

Catastrophizing

You overestimate the chances of disaster. You anticipate the worst.

> "My back pain is getting worse. I know I'll need surgery, and my life will nevver be the same again."

> "I'll be stuck forever in this traffic jam, the meeting will go on without me, and I'll end up getting fired."

> "I forgot to pay this bill. My credit rating will drop, all my credit cards will be canceled, and my finances will be in tatters."

Minimizing or Disqualifying the Positive

You discount the positive in a situation and undervalue your accomplishments.

> "I made the deadline, but anyone could do that."

> "Even with my bad back, I was able to do the water aerobics class for the first time. It was no big deal. The pool was filled with older people."

> "I solved the problem, but they would have figured it out on their own."

Maximizing or Filtering

You exaggerate the importance of one negative event and disregard the good.

> "So what if people praised my new recipe. My tennis partner found it too salty. I can't make that again."

> "My evaluation said I was doing a great job, but one manager said I could be more enthusiastic. I'm never going to measure up."

"My back was so bad I couldn't pick up my grandson. It was terrible. Even if my physical therapist says my spine is getting more flexible, I don't see it."

Personalizing

You automatically blame yourself when something bad happens, even if you were not responsible.

"If it hadn't been for me, the team would have won the championship."

"If only I had warned her, she would never have dated the guy who broke her heart."

"If only I didn't encourage him to take up golf, he never would have developed back problems."

Mind Reading

You baselessly believe that someone is reacting badly to you and do nothing to verify your conclusion.

"My boss looked at his phone during my presentation. He thinks I am boring."

"I can tell he doesn't care about me."

"They all think I'm exaggerating my back problems to avoid working on the group project."

Fortune Telling

You predict what will happen on little evidence.

"There is no point in even trying. It's not going to work."

"I know no one will show up for the party. It's going to be a flop."

"I just know my back will get worse and ruin the vacation I've been looking forward to."

All or Nothing Thinking

You see things as either good or bad, black or white. There is no middle ground. If you are not perfect, you are a total failure.

"I never get what I want."

"Nothing ever works to make me feel better."

"I always make a mess of things."

Overgeneralizing

You see a single negative event as a pattern of defeat that will not end.

"She didn't want to meet for a drink. No one wants to spend time with me."

"I have had a setback. I know I will never make it back to normal no matter what I do."

"You are never ready on time. We're always late for everything."

Emotional Reasoning

You accept your emotions as fact and do not think logically. You assume your negative emotions reflect the way things really are. If you feel something, it must be true.

"I am afraid of public speaking. I will never be able to deliver a good toast."

"I feel anxious, so I know something terrible is going to happen."

"I feel hopeless. This program will never work."

Should Statements

You attempt to motivate yourself with should and shouldn't, must and ought. The emotional consequence is guilt. If you direct the "shoulds" at others, you end up angry, frustrated, and resentful.

"I should have been promoted to vice president by now."

"I should push myself harder during my daily workouts."

"He should pay more attention to me."

Labeling and Mislabeling

This is an extreme form of generalization, which involves attaching a label.

"I'm an idiot. I can never remember his name."

"He's such a loser. He never comes through."

"I'm a cripple. This back pain has made my life miserable."

If you have heard a playback loop in your head with repetitive thoughts like these examples of negative distortions—and just about everyone has—now is the time to break those negative thought patterns and make a shift to the bright side.

ABCD FOR IDENTIFYING AND RESTRUCTURING YOUR SELF-DEFEATING THINKING PATTERNS

The field of Cognitive Behavioral Therapy (CBT), founded by Aaron T. Beck, emphasizes that negative thought patterns can have a profound effect on your physical and mental well-being by raising stress levels that contribute to anxiety and depression. Psychologist Albert Ellis first introduced the ABCD model to help people overcome pessimistic thinking. The process involves identifying self-defeating thinking habits, challenging them logically, and replacing them with more helpful and realistic thinking. The ABCD model will help you to practice restructuring your thoughts to create ones that are more balanced, realistic, and helpful. To restructure an automatic thought pattern, apply the ABCD model, an illustration of which follows:

A. **Antecedent (trigger or event)**

Speaking in public

B. Beliefs (automatic thoughts)

"I am just too nervous to give a speech at the conference. It will be a disaster."

C. Consequences (resulting feeling and behaviors)

Anxiety, self-doubt, fear of failure

D. Dispute (challenging the negative thoughts)

"This is an opportunity to overcome this fear. If I want to rise in my profession, I have to get over this. I have plenty of time to prepare and practice."

The more you practice noticing your automatic thoughts, the better able you will be to decide which need to be restructured. By slowing down and examining your thinking, you can edit your negative thoughts and select the ones that are supportive of you and what you are doing.

I have made a table of negative thoughts and their positive counterparts to give you examples of how to respond to the world with positivity. You can apply the ABCD model to the distorted negative thinking in the chart that follows to understand how the positive thoughts evolved. Soon you will realize that growth comes from noticing and editing your negative thoughts. Doing so will change your world.

CONVERTING NEGATIVE THINKING TO POSITIVE THINKING

Negative Thought	Positive Thought
I always mess up.	I do many things well.
I'm a failure.	I made a mistake, which is an opportunity to learn and grow.

I'm having a breakdown.	This could be a breakthrough-in-progress.
I'm not as lucky as other people.	Good things can and will happen to me.
I don't think I will . . .	I am confident that . . .
I should be better than I am.	I am making an effort to improve.
If only . . .	Next time . . .
It's a problem.	It's an opportunity.
I'm not smart enough.	I am smart in my own way and can learn.
I am worried that I won't do well.	I know that with effort I can do well.
I never win.	I tried hard, improved, and achieved a lot.
It's too complicated.	I'll tackle it from a different angle.
I'm worried that I will let others down.	I will try hard and do my best.
I'm not going to get better at this.	I will give it another try.
Life's a struggle.	Life's an adventure.
I ate all those cookies. I'll never lose weight.	One setback is not the end of the world. I'll get right back on track.
I will never get it right.	I will try something different next time.
I have to exercise.	I get to exercise.

As long as you go about your life with a negative inner dialogue, you are supporting those existing patterns in your brain. What you think, feel, imagine, and pay attention to shapes your brain through a process called neuroplasticity. When you repeat a negative thought pattern again and again, the connections between the neurons in your brain strengthen, and that type of thinking becomes automatic, called negative neuroplasticity. The good news is that your brain has the capacity to reorganize pathways, create new connections, and in some cases, generate new neurons, called positive neuroplasticity. Science has found that the brain is far more flexible than previously believed, and that it accepts drastic changes in mindset. The good news is that repeated, regular, positive thinking, and acting in a positive manner can re-wire your brain and make it stronger. In time, you can change how you naturally think and change your life for the better as a result. It takes commitment and work to mold your brain and to transform the way you respond to the world. Engaging in more positive thinking will help you to handle the stress in your life and consequently will reduce your pain.

AFFIRMATIONS

Affirmations are short, powerful statements that allow you to be in control of your thoughts. These positive declarations help your mind to prioritize positivity over negativity. I am listing some examples to inspire you. I hope you will create your own affirmations to reflect your needs and desires. You should make affirmations a part of your daily life. Think them, say them, and write them down.

I can and I will.

I deserve everything my good life has to offer.

I always keep promises I make to myself.

I refuse to give up because I haven't tried all possible ways.

I don't sweat the small stuff.

I am good and getting better.

I am in charge of how I feel, and today I am choosing brave.

I am enough.

I treat everyone with respect and care, as I want to be treated.

I have the power to create change.

Life does not have to be perfect to be wonderful.

I am in the right place at the right time.

Being happy is productive.

I can do this.

I will stop holding on to what hurts and make room for what feels good.

I love taking responsibility for my life.

I'm open-minded and accept people as they are.

I'm so grateful for the little things that put a smile on my face.

It's a good day to have a good day.

Courage starts with showing up.

This is the perfect moment.

I will do things I think I cannot do.

I'm getting stronger every day.

I choose what I become.

Everything is temporary.

Perfection is a myth.

I'm ready enough.

HOW TO TRAIN YOUR MIND TO BE MORE POSITIVE

There are many things you can do to change the tone of your inner voice from self-criticism to self-acceptance, from doom and gloom to enthusiasm and wholehearted participation in life. Think of your beautiful mind as its own inner environment. Reflect on the types of thoughts you want living there. What kinds of ideas do you want to guide your life? You would want supportive thoughts that make you more resilient in the face of stress. You would choose thoughts that reflect the direction you want to be going and let go of the ingrained thoughts that keep you stuck where you have been. You have the power to make that choice and rid yourself of self-defeating negativity.

The first step in waking up from an automatic life is paying attention:

- Your work begins with becoming aware of the patterns of your thoughts, feelings, and reactions as they happen. In other words, be mindful of what your inner voice is saying.

- As you listen to the tape that always plays in your head, identify the areas in your life that trigger negative thoughts. Is it work, a relationship, or a type of situation?

- Challenge your inner critic. Evaluate negative thoughts rationally. Remind yourself that thoughts or feelings are not always reality. Consider whether the thought is a fact or an opinion, whether the thinking is helping or hurting you.

- As you look at your thoughts, shift your perspective by stepping back. Are you assigning too much importance to the situation that is bothering you? Will it matter in one week? In one year? In five years?

- Reframe the thought. Consciously put a positive spin on the negative thought.

- Stop and check yourself during the day and evaluate what you are thinking. Replace negative thoughts with something better. If the negativity is very strong, go for neutrality.

With practice, you will learn to quiet the negative chatter in your head and train your brain to respond to situations calmly, rationally, and optimistically. If you dedicate yourself to changing the way you see the world, your life will be fuller and richer with so much to distract you from your pain.

HOW TO ENHANCE YOUR POSITIVITY

Certain daily rituals can foster positivity and remind you of your goal. Consider these daily practices exercise for your brain:

- Start the day with a positive affirmation and repeat it ten times.

- Try to keep your focus on the present, the exact moment, here and now.

- Be thankful for what and who you have.

- Keep a gratitude journal.

- Be kind to yourself.

- Find humor in any situation.

- Remember the good moments, no matter how small, and savor them.

- If your inner voice is saying something you would not say to your best friend, banish the idea from your mind or edit it.

- Turn failures and disappointments into lessons.

- Collect inspirational quotes and share them with friends.

- Surround yourself with positive people. They can inspire you with their example. Some of their positivity just might rub off.

- Help someone. Small acts of kindness feel good.

- Set a goal you can attain and record your progress.
- Make sure you have some time each day to do something you enjoy. It can be as little as five minutes.

I am sure you can add many things to this list that will make you feel good about your life. Any one of these actions will lift your spirits and set you on the path to positivity.

PAIN AND NEGATIVITY

The experience of pain is much more complicated than just the physical perception of pain. The longer you suffer from back pain, the less it has to do with the original physical problem and the more it is linked to your emotional state. Chronic pain adds another layer to your negative thoughts, which can wreck your quality of life. If you are in pain, you must work harder to stay positive. If you are able to overcome the negativity pain can generate, you will be in a better position to cope with your pain. The remainder of this chapter will show you how to react to and transform your thought patterns to foster a sense of control over your life.

WHAT BUTTONS PAIN CAN PUSH IN YOUR THINKING

I do not have to tell you that dealing with chronic back pain is frustrating and exhausting. It goes beyond physical discomfort. You also have to cope with the enervating psychological and emotional side of living with pain. Pain catastrophizing is a common thinking pattern that accompanies chronic pain. The negative thoughts of this pattern contribute to how you perceive the intensity of your pain and the emotional distress it is causing you.

People with chronic pain tend to magnify the power of their pain and to worry that the pain will get worse. Pain can become their worst enemy.

That magnification can lead to a feeling of helplessness and lack of control. They doubt their ability to cope. They worry that their unbearable pain will never end. Chronic pain changes people's lives. If their mobility is restricted, pain can seem to shrink their lives. A sense of loss creeps into their thoughts.

Psychologists use the term rumination to describe another mode of thinking people with pain can fall into. Rumination involves continuously thinking about the pain, which can consume so much time and energy that their pain dominates their thoughts. There is no room for anything else in their minds. Rumination focuses on the symptoms without thoughts of doing something about it. Magnification, rumination, and feelings of helplessness and loss are stress magnifiers, and you know what that means. Experiencing more stress will only raise the level of inflammation in your body, a formula for pain.

These examples of pain catastrophizing demonstrate the negative rut the minds of pain sufferers can get stuck in:

Magnification

"I'm afraid the pain will get worse."

"Something serious must be causing the pain."

"I find myself thinking of other painful events, and this is the worst."

Helplessness

"I can't take it anymore."

"The pain is awful, it's overwhelming."

"I feel I can't go on."

"I think it's never going to get better."

"Nothing helps. Nothing I do works to reduce the intensity of the pain."

Rumination

"I keep thinking about how badly I want the pain to stop."

"I cannot keep the pain out of my mind."

"It hurts so much it's all I can think of."

"All I can think of is wanting the pain to go away."

"I worry all the time about whether the pain will ever end."

I have heard these words, or ones like them, countless times from patients. I explain to them that these thoughts are doing nothing to improve their condition, that negativity is making them feel worse. I assure them that viewing their pain differently will help them rise above their suffering.

PUTTING A POSITIVE SPIN ON YOUR NEGATIVE THOUGHTS ABOUT PAIN

You can change your negative mindset in response to your pain, just as you can change a negative worldview. It is a matter of shifting your perspective. The chart that follows illustrates how to turn a negative thought about pain and its effects on your life into one that is practical, hopeful, and empowering.

Negative	Positive
There must be something seriously wrong with me because the pain is bad.	Back pain does not have to be caused by damage or injury.
I've tried everything. Nothing can help my pain.	Though I can't find a medical solution, I will learn coping skills to manage the pain.
It hurts when I do things.	I would rather do things and hurt than not do things and still hurt. Moving is good for me.

I'm in so much pain, I'm not getting out of bed until I feel better.	I'll get up to take care of my basic needs. By using my pain-management tools and the Watch Your Back program, I will be up and around soon.
I never have the energy to do everything I want to.	I can learn to pace myself to accomplish things.
I just can't handle the pain.	Not every day is a bad day. I can get through this. Better days are ahead.
I'll never get any sleep, so I won't make it through the day.	I can use the sleepless time to rest. No matter how much sleep I get, I can still function tomorrow. I can nap and catch up tomorrow night.
I can't do anything anymore.	I may not be able to do all I used to do, but I can still be happy and live well despite the pain. The Watch Your Back program will expand my horizons.
If I go to the gym, I'll have pain for days to pay for it.	I can do stretches and gentle exercise instead of pushing too hard. I'll make note of a workout's exercises, intensity, and duration to learn what crosses the line and causes a flare-up.
My life is a mess.	I have it better than many other people. Things could be a lot worse.
I don't think I can go on like this.	I'm not a quitter. No matter what happens, I'll make it. I am not hopeless.

Acceptance and Commitment

You have learned how to examine and restructure your thoughts, but some thoughts can be persistent and hard to change. Sometimes if you challenge the content and accuracy of your automatic negative thoughts and interpretations, you can feel even more distressed. If you try to change those thoughts, you can make them stronger. The more attention you pay to some thoughts, the stronger they become.

Acceptance and Commitment Therapy (ACT) is another approach to dealing with negativity, developed by Steven C. Hayes, that is particularly effective with chronic pain. The focus in CBT (Cognitive Behavioral Therapy) is on challenging and changing distorted thoughts, while the focus of ACT is on being aware and nonjudgmental of your thoughts. The shift is from changing negative thoughts, to recognizing thoughts as just thoughts, no more and no less. With ACT, you learn to become present with your patterns of thinking in a broader, more flexible way.

We all tend to identify with our thoughts, amplifying them in our minds to the status of facts and the truth. If you become accustomed to viewing your thoughts this way, they can control you and prevent you from seeing other options. The aim of Acceptance and Commitment Therapy is to allow you to get some distance from your thoughts, so that you can recognize them for what they are. When you observe a thought, you can see how it structures your world, but you understand that you are the one who is doing the structuring. With this technique, you develop a different awareness and relationship to your thoughts. You notice, distance, and disconnect from your thoughts and feelings. You see them for what they are: streams of words, passing sensations, and not what the voice inside is saying they are—unequivocal facts and inescapable dangers. When you stop, step back, and observe thoughts and feelings without judging, you deactivate or neutralize them.

Though Acceptance and Commitment Therapy focuses on willingly accepting some pain without judgment, the end goal is not just to accept your situation. Part of the process is identifying values that align with your goals for your life and committing to pursuing them. When it comes to pain, ACT operates from the belief that pain itself is not the source of suffering, rather the psychological struggle of dealing with the pain is the challenge.

Cognitive Distancing

Cognitive distancing, known in psychological terms as cognitive defusion, is a process developed by Dr. Aaron Beck. With this technique, you establish a different relationship with the stream of thoughts that flows through your head all the time. Your mind naturally labels, categorizes, dissects, compares, and evaluates just about everything you experience. Negative judgments can become your reality when your mind fuses those thoughts with direct experience so that you do not distinguish between the two. The thoughts themselves are not the problem, your fusion with those thoughts is.

When you practice cognitive defusion, you will:

- Achieve more distance from negative thoughts.

- Observe your thoughts rather than being swept up by them.

- See that your thoughts often do not correspond with reality. This perception will result in taking these thoughts less seriously.

- Increase your focus on direct experiences, such as feelings, observations, and sensations.

In your new relationship with negative thinking, you do not try to suppress the troubling thoughts that pop into your head, but neither do you defer to them. You determine what thoughts will help you solve problems and will take you in the direction you want to go. You evaluate if a set of thoughts will enable you to live a rich life or if they are creating needless pain. Cognitive defusion gets you out of your head and into direct experience.

By viewing thoughts as thoughts, you lessen the impact of long-standing thinking patterns without having to change the content of those thoughts. You let the thoughts come and go. When you are dealing with chronic pain, this technique allows you to shift your focus from reducing and eliminating pain to engaging fully in your life.

PASSENGERS ON THE BUS

If cognitive defusion seems too abstract to you, there is a classic exercise that explains the process:

Imagine your life is like driving a bus. There are passengers on the bus, and you are picking up more. Think of the passengers as everything that goes on inside you, your thoughts, feelings, beliefs, sensations, memories, fantasies. The road represents the outside world, the situations, and people you encounter.

Some of the passengers are benign, but many of them are bullies. They do not hesitate to speak up and criticize you. Then they become real back seat drivers, telling you how to drive and where to go.

So, what do you do? You could tell them to quiet down or argue with them. You could stop the bus and try to reason with them. If you do that, you are no longer driving the bus. You are dealing with them. All your energy is spent arguing with the passengers rather than getting where you want to go. Some of the passengers won't listen to reason. They are very pushy. They demand that you do what they say.

You could try to make peace with the bullies. You could give in because it is too hard to stand up to them. It may feel safer to go along with the passengers in the short term, but you are not moving toward your destination.

The fact is that you are the driver of the bus. You may not be able to make the passengers keep quiet, but they cannot make you do anything. Are you going to follow their directions or continue to try to control them? Or are you going to drive the bus, making the stops you want to make, moving toward your destination?

This story is a metaphor for dealing with your inner voice, for not letting negative thought patterns keep you from leading the life you want to live.

TECHNIQUES FOR DISTANCING YOURSELF FROM YOUR THOUGHTS

You can use cognitive distancing techniques on repetitive, self-sabotaging thoughts at any time as they stream through your mind, or you can focus on a single, troubling, self-critical thought. If you choose to focus on one negative thought that troubles you, follow these steps:

- Think about the negative thought you have about yourself.

- Condense that story into a short phrase, for example, "I'm an idiot," "I'm a loser," "Nobody likes me."

- Concentrate on that phrase for a minute or two, which will create a sense of fusion with the tag.

- Then you can use that troubling self-evaluation as the target for practicing defusion techniques.

To deal with a self-defeating thought, try the techniques that follow.

"I Notice . . ."

Add the phrase "I notice I am having the thought that . . ." or simply, "I'm having the thought that . . ." at the start of your recurring negative thoughts. For example, "I notice I am having the thought that the pain will never go away."

By using the "I notice" point of view whenever negative thoughts pop into your mind, you will begin to change your relationship with that thought. You will put distance between the thought and yourself. You will no longer fuse your identity with that unhelpful judgment.

Give Your Negative Thoughts a Name

You can give a name to a recurring thought, for instance, "I notice I'm having my 'I can't do it' thought," or "There it is again, my 'I can't take it anymore' thought." Once again, you are putting space between you and that thought.

"Thank You, Mind"

With this technique, you do not take your negative thoughts too seriously. When an unhelpful thought arises, you thank your mind sarcastically. "Thanks a lot for that fascinating thought . . ." or "Thanks for the feedback . . ." or "Thanks for that . . ." Your mental tone is dismissive. The goal is to change your relationship to that thought.

Repeating the Thought

Repeat a negative thought—"you fool," for example—out loud in slow motion, using a funny voice, or singing the thought out loud and over and over until it loses meaning and only the sound remains. Does the thought lose its power when you do any of these things? Does it make you as uncomfortable as it did before you practiced this technique?

Pop-Up Mind

Imagine that your unhelpful thought is an internet pop-up ad. Imagine clicking to close the window.

Practice Mindful Watching

Pay attention to your thoughts with an open, accepting, and curious manner without trying to control or manage them. The following chapter on mindfulness meditation will expand on this practice.

I hope you are feeling more upbeat after reading these pages. Knowing that you are in control of what you think can be liberating. This chapter has given you ways to reframe negative thinking and to distance yourself from automatic thoughts that are holding you back and intensifying your pain. At the same time, you have learned how to distance yourself from the psychological effects of pain. The next chapter will examine mindfulness and meditation as a means to calming both your mind and body.

Chapter 12

Strategy 9:
Meditation to the Rescue

Meditation takes mindfulness to a new level. The previous chapter introduced you to Cognitive Behavioral Therapy (CBT) and Acceptance and Commitment Therapy (ACT), methods of dealing with your endlessly chattering inner voice. The aim of the first technique is to observe and replace negative thoughts with positive ones, and the second is to observe and commit to embracing more realistic self-talk. Mindfulness meditation, a part of Jon Kabat-Zinn's Mindfulness-Based Stress Reduction program, involves being consciously aware of and committed to staying in the now.

When you meditate, you pay attention to your thoughts, feelings, sensations, and emotions without judgments or criticism. Mindfulness means observing the moment without being stuck in the past or worried about the future. The objective is not to clear your mind of thoughts or to achieve an out-of-body experience. You do not alter or detach from your thoughts. Instead, you pay attention to the present with full conscious awareness and notice when your mind wanders off. You become present and awake at the point between the past and the future. Meditation is a workout for your brain. It helps you to balance thoughts of the past, present, and future.

THE POWER OF MEDITATION

Arjun, an international entrepreneur, always traveled first class. He ate all the meals offered on his international flights, watched all the movies, and drank the complimentary alcohol. Arjun smoked a pack per day. At 5 feet 11 inches, he weighed 245 pounds with a BMI of 34. He was obese. Arjun's conglomeration of businesses was in financial trouble, and he was under a good deal of stress.

After we met at a conference in Toronto, Arjun came to New York to evaluate his neck pain. An MRI scan showed a herniation on his left side C6-C7. Thinking that surgery was the only way, Arjun panicked. He could not afford to be out of commission. His international consortium of companies demanded his full attention.

I introduced Arjun to the principles of Watch Your Back. He started by avoiding bending, lifting, twisting, and reaching to calm down the nerves of his spine. He began taking gabapentin at night to help the nerve root pain and an anti-inflammatory in the morning. We immediately arranged physical therapy treatments during his stay in New York. One week later, Arjun was much better. The edge was off his neck pain.

I encouraged him to walk daily. He set a goal of losing fifty pounds in a year. One pound a week seemed achievable to him. "I can do that easily," Arjun said.

He gave up his three drinks a day and did not miss them. He did not need a drink after a long day because he had started to meditate, which was a great stress reliever and would contribute significantly to weight loss. In the course of one year, he stopped smoking. He was determined to stay healthy. He had to take care of himself if he wanted to run a successful business.

Arjun had no trouble embracing the strategies of good posture, deep belly breathing, spinal range of motion, and spinal strengthening. He meditated each day and had a life-changing breakthrough while meditating. The thought came to him that "my children are my children, and my businesses are not my children." Inspired by this insight, Arjun started to reorganize his business, selling or closing any business that did not provide income. He regularly met and networked with India's most outstanding business minds.

With his business back on track, it did not take long for Arjun to feel better, lighter, and happier. Once his weight was down, he hired a running coach and committed to training for a marathon. Though I usually do not recommend high impact aerobics for patients with back problems, Arjun's trouble spot was his neck. I have seen that many of my patients with neck problems feel better when they run. In one year, Arjun was lightweight, fit, and pain free. He is wafer-thin at 170 pounds and has a BMI of 24.

On his first-class flights these days, Arjun consumes a hefty 16-ounce bottle of water, nuts, and healthy snacks. He also makes sure to get up from his seat every hour. To help avoid jet lag and to get the restorative sleep he needs, this world traveler uses his soft silicone earplugs and his 3D contoured cup sleeping mask and blindfold. During the flight, he falls asleep on his extended, full-length bed and never forgets to put up his Do Not Disturb sign.

With a dream, a dare, determination, and discipline to improve his life, Arjun achieved excellent results. Arjun runs an international company today.

THE FAR-REACHING BENEFITS OF MEDITATION

Studies of mindful meditation have found surprising benefits. Research has shown that practicing meditation regularly lowers blood pressure, heart-rate, and brain activity. Remember neuroplasticity? Brain imaging studies have revealed that meditation can physically change brain regions linked to memory, sense of self, and brain activity. Other studies extend that influence on areas of the brain responsible for focus, body awareness, memory, emotional regulation, and communication.

Several recent studies have shown that meditation can change your genes. Specifically, meditation lowers levels of pro-inflammatory genes. The down-regulation of those genes provides a faster recovery from stressful situations. A 2017 Harvard Medical School study found that meditating for fifteen minutes a day for eight weeks changed 172 genes that control inflammation, sleep-wake rhythms, and how your body processes sugar, all of which play a role in chronic pain. Meditation reduces cognitive stress and the physical arousal it causes and increases positive states of mind.

Meditation also has an anti-aging effect. Harvard scientists examined the markers of aging in cells of a group who had started to meditate. They measured telomeres, protective protein caps at the end of DNA strands. The study also looked at telomerase, an enzyme that helps to protect and lengthen those DNA caps. As you age, chronic stress causes the protein caps in your DNA to unravel, resulting in shorter chromosomes and aging cells. The longer your telomere caps are the more times a cell can regenerate, which extends your lifespan.

In addition, the length of your telomeres is related to how well your immune system and cardiovascular system work. Cells die fast and are more prone to disease with shorter telomeres. Meditation reduces the effects of stress on your telomeres, keeping them from unraveling. Science has shown that meditation can help to keep your cells healthier and younger, a benefit that will enhance your overall sense of well-being.

INFLAMMATORY STRESS

John is a forty-year-old executive, who had been experiencing stiffness in his thoracic spine. His lower back did not bother him as much. John's work life was a bit out of control. He was working sixty hours a week. He was under so much pressure that he was not eating well. He had no time to exercise, and he tossed and turned every night in bed.

Even then, his main complaint was stiffness, an inability to bend his spine. He moved his whole body like a wooden soldier. His neck, back, and lower back were immobile.

X-rays revealed bone formation called bridging on the front of his vertebrae, the weight-bearing part of vertebrae. His rheumatologist diagnosed ankylosing spondylitis based on his X-rays. John was well along with his disease, with vertebral bone to bone showing fusion throughout his spine. Ankylosing spondylitis is an inflammatory disease that usually begins in early adulthood. The disease reduces the spine's flexibility. Patients with this condition become increasingly kyphotic in the thoracic spine, which means an exaggerated forward rounding of the upper back and a hunch forward. A blood test revealed that his C-reactive protein, an inflammatory marker, was elevated at 10, the start of what is considered a high level.

John wanted to deal with the disease before it became worse. He came to see me for a consultation. As we discussed his situation, I suggested that he view his back problem as an opportunity to improve his overall health.

He knew he had to take better care of himself, or his health would decline. If he wanted to extend his working life, he would have to make some changes. He learned to manage his time better to fit exercise into his busy schedule. He had to develop a better bedtime routine to relax and unwind rather than fretting about what had gone on that day or what was in store for him the next day. Mindful meditation helped him to calm down and not to overreact to every slight annoyance.

In two years, John was feeling much better about himself. I worked with John to strengthen his core muscles. John started with the strengthening Watch Your Back Workout 1, consisting of Pelvic Tilting, Knee-to-Chest Hug, Cat-Cow stretch, Bridge work, Hamstring Stretches with Towel, and the Cobra position. Within a few months John switched to the second Watch Your Back Workout, which includes the Corner Stretch, Lying Lateral Leg Lifts, Plank, Supine Trunk Rotation, Bird Dog, and Child's Pose.

John took up gentle, progressive yoga being careful always to never stretch beyond his comfort level. He grew more flexible. He had abundant energy and was more relaxed. The range of motion in his neck, back, pelvis, hips, knees, ankles, and feet had improved. John told me that he had discovered a new range of motion in his eyes. If he is feeling negative, he looks down. When John is happy, his gaze is up and rising. He said he wanted to keep looking up.

MEDITATION AND BACK PAIN

I suggest that you try a short daily meditation, which will be an effective tool for reducing your back pain. Meditation produces powerful, pain-relieving effects in the brain. One study, published in the *Journal of Neuroscience*, found about a 40 percent reduction in pain intensity and a 57 percent reduction in pain unpleasantness in subjects who meditated. Meditation produced a greater reduction in pain than morphine or other pain-relieving drugs, which typically reduce pain ratings by 25 percent.

Imaging studies of the brain show that mindfulness soothes the brain patterns underlying pain. Over time, these changes alter the structure of the brain itself. As a result, you no longer feel the pain with the same intensity. Functional MRIs confirm that people who suffer from chronic pain have more brain tissue dedicated to handling the conscious sensations of pain. It is as if the volume of pain is turned up to maximum, and the brain cannot turn it down. Mindfulness meditation allows you to control how loud your pain is in your mind. A study done at the Group Health Research Institute in Seattle, Washington, published in the *Journal of the American Medical Association*, found that meditation improved the ability to perform daily activities like walking, climbing stairs, and standing in subjects with chronic pain by 60 percent.

One way that meditation can help to ease your pain is by moving your attention away from the pain. The focus is on becoming aware of body sensations, thoughts, and emotions without trying to change them. As you meditate, your muscle tension and heart rate drop, your respiration slows, and your breath gets deeper. The relaxing aspect of meditation helps to unclench back muscles.

Mindfulness meditation improves your ability to pay attention to the present moment while you maintain an accepting, nonjudgmental awareness of what you are experiencing in that moment. Mindfulness will help you to put some space between yourself and your reactions, and that distance can break down your conditioned responses to pain.

The aim of meditation is not to quiet your mind or to try to achieve a state of internal calm. The goal is simply to pay attention to the present moment without judgment. When you notice that judgments arise while you are meditating, let them roll by. Make a mental note of them and let them pass. Return to observing the present moment as it is. Your mind might often get carried away in thought. Mindfulness meditation is the practice of returning, again and again, to the present moment. Do not judge yourself for whatever thoughts crop up. Just recognize that your mind has wandered off and gently bring it back. It sounds simple, but you will probably not find it as easy as it sounds. It takes practice.

BASIC MINDFUL MEDITATION

This simple meditation focuses on the breath because the physical sensation of breathing is always there, and you can use it as an anchor to the present moment. While you are meditating, you may find yourself caught up in thoughts, emotions, sounds. Wherever your mind goes, simply come back to the next breath.

You do not have to meditate for hours to benefit from mindful meditation. If you are just starting out, aim for five to ten minutes every day. If you are too restless and find meditation too challenging, try being still for just one minute. When you can sit and relax that long, increase your meditation time to two minutes and continue to increase the time as you get comfortable meditating. The important thing is to start. The length of time you spend meditating will grow naturally. Find the amount of time that works for you and do it every day. Many studies suggest that fifteen to twenty minutes of mindfulness meditation per day can result in significant benefits, but you can feel a difference when you meditate for just five to ten minutes a day. For maximum impact, meditating for twenty minutes twice a day is recommended.

When you sit to meditate, you can set a timer or an alarm rather than wondering how much time is left. Knowing that you do not have to worry when your session will end can help you stay in the present.

How to Meditate

As you learn how to meditate, you should find a quiet place to avoid distractions. Try not to drink a caffeinated beverage before meditation because you do not need extra stimulation when you are trying to relax. Avoid meditating soon after a meal if you do not want your meditation session to turn into a nap.

- Using a cushion or comfortable chair in a quiet place, sit up straight with your hands on your lap. Close your eyes.

- Allow your body to be still. Feel as if you are sinking into the chair.

- Take two or three deep breaths. Notice your increased sense of calm.

- Begin to breathe naturally. Feel the air enter your nose, move through your throat, and enter your lungs as your stomach expands and falls back down again.

- Focus on your breath. You might want to think the words "in" and "out" as you breathe.

- As thoughts or feelings arise, observe them as they come and go as if you are watching a movie.

- If you become distracted by a thought, gently turn your attention away from the thought and return it to your breathing. Some people count their breaths to remain focused.

- Do not be critical of yourself if your mind wanders off and rests on a thought. Just return your focus to your breath.

- When you are ready to end your session, bring your attention back into your body and the room. Move around gently in the chair.

- Open your eyes and stretch out.

MINDFUL MEDITATION HURDLES

Focusing on the here and now is harder than it sounds. Several tricks of the mind can interfere with meditating. I am mentioning them so that you will recognize these common obstacles to practicing mindfulness.

> **Restlessness:** Staying still might be a challenge for you, and meditation might seem boring. If that is the case, try focusing on specific sensations, like exhaling. You can make your exhalations longer than inhalations. Do not be hard on yourself. Just bring yourself back to the present moment.

> **Self-criticism:** When you begin to meditate, be prepared to experience some self-doubt. "I'm doing it all wrong" or "I'll never be a good meditator" are common forms of self-criticism. Try to let go of any judgments you might have of what is good meditation or bad meditation, and whether you are achieving anything. Remember: everyone has the capacity for clarity, calm, and mindfulness.

> **Sleepiness:** Many people get sleepy when they try to meditate. When you are feeling drowsy, there are several ways you can wake yourself up. You can straighten your posture or open your eyes. Instead of focusing on your breath, try shifting your attention, for example, to sounds.

> **Pain:** Whether it is aches in your back or cramps in your legs, notice the pain and accept it. Acknowledge that it is a feeling like any other feeling, and you can choose to pay attention to it or not. Notice the pain, pause, and then come back to the present moment.

> **Fear:** Panic or fear can arise when you meditate. If that occurs, shift your attention to something outside your body like the sound of the air going in and out of your nostrils. Do not pay close attention to what might be causing your emotional response. If it becomes intense, open your eyes and take a break.

MINI-MEDITATIONS

A quick meditation can calm you down if you are having a meltdown or acute reaction to something. Just a minute of mindful meditation can shift your focus. You can use mini-meditations anywhere and anytime you need to pause and to come back to your calm self. Using this technique will save you from the wear and tear of daily stress.

For pain flare-ups:

- Pause for a moment instead of automatically reacting to the pain.

- Observe what is happening that moment in your body and mind, your thoughts, emotions, and sensations.

- Focus on how breathing feels, the air moving into your nostrils and your belly rising and falling with each breath.

- Expand your awareness to your body and mind.

- Make a mindful decision about what to do next instead of reacting automatically.

For stress:

- Stop and notice the physical signs of your stress response. Are your fists clenched? Are you grinding your teeth? Are you breathing shallowly? Is your mind galloping? Identify what your body does in response to stress.

- Consider these actions a cue that you need to relax.

- Simply noticing that you are stressed can make you realize you have a choice about what to do about it.

For anxiety:

When anxious thoughts strike, you have a ninety-second window to intervene before you set off a stress reaction that might take a lot more time to recover from, both physically and emotionally. Use this shortcut to mindfulness to quiet your anxiety.

If stressful thoughts are building into a big reaction, imagine a "clear button" at the center of your palm. Press the button with the index finger of your opposite hand. Keep pressing it as you picture it signaling your stress response to calm down. Count slowly to three, taking a deep breath with each count. On your final exhale, let go of the anxious feelings and come back to the present moment. If one try doesn't help, repeat the process two or three times until it works.

WALKING MEDITATION

You do not have to do your meditations sitting still. Walking meditation is a variant of standard mindful meditation you might want to try if you are having difficulty with seated meditation, or you just want to switch it up. This moving meditation can give your body a rest from your sitting posture. If your body becomes achy and irritable from sitting meditation, you might want to give it a try.

Working with the sensation of breathing as a focus does not do the trick for everyone. Sometimes the sensation of breath is not enough to keep your mind from wandering. Focusing on how the soles of your feet feel as you walk can be more concrete and accessible.

Walking meditation is just what it sounds like. It is based on your walking gait. It is a reflection of something you do regularly, except you slow it down. Practicing walking meditation gives you the chance to tune in anytime you feel stiff or sore, overwhelmed or ungrounded. During walking meditation, you place your attention far from your thinking mind to your feet, a physical gap between thinking and feeling. Walking meditation is about being aware of your body and physical sensations as you move.

The recommendation is to do ten minutes a day for at least a week. Mindfulness is said to increase the more you practice this meditation.

- You can practice walking meditation outside or indoors. You can choose to move in a circle, back and forth, or in a straight line.

Practicing indoors may be a good option because you can focus directly on mindfulness with fewer opportunities to be distracted by your surroundings. If you walk in a public space, make sure you will not get in the way of others.

- Find a space or lane that allows you to walk back and forth for ten to fifteen paces or in a circle without obstacles. You will not have a destination, so if you choose to move back and forth the lane does not have to be very long. If you are outside, you will not have to walk back and forth. The place where you practice walking meditation outside should be quiet without a lot of traffic because slow, formal walking can look strange to people who do not know what you are doing.

- Anchor yourself by taking a few deep breaths as you bring your full attention to your body. Be aware of how stable the ground feels beneath your feet. Take note of the sensations in your body and your thoughts and feelings.

- Walk ten to fifteen steps along the route you have chosen. Pay attention to the movement of your feet and legs. Try not to be mechanical or rigid as you walk. Keep your body upright and aligned. Pause and breathe for as long as you like after you take ten to fifteen steps.

- If you are meditating indoors, turn and walk back in the opposite direction, retracing your steps. Otherwise, continue walking along your path.

- If you are pacing back and forth, turn again and continue the walk.

- The meditation involves deliberate thinking about doing a series of actions that you do automatically.

- Breaking your steps down in your mind may seem odd, but you will train yourself to notice four basic components of each step you take:

  1. Lift the back of your foot off the ground.

  2. Observe your back foot as it swings forward and lowers.

3. Observe your back foot as it makes contact with the ground, heel first.

4. Feel the weight shift onto the foot as the body moves forward.

- You can walk at any speed. The recommendation is to walk slowly and to take small steps. The movements should feel natural, not exaggerated.

- Your arms can hang at your sides, or you can clasp them in back or in front of you.

- As you walk, focus your attention on one or more sensations that you normally take for granted, the movement of your feet and legs, their contact with the floor or ground, your breath coming in and out of your body, sounds nearby or caused by your body's movement, or what your eyes take in as you focus on what is in front of you.

- Inevitably, your mind will wander. When you notice the wandering, bring your attention back to focus on one of the sensations you are experiencing.

Though walking meditation may seem strange at first, it will grow on you. You can bring mindfulness to walking at any speed, even running. In time, you will be able to bring the same degree of awareness to any everyday activity. The goal is to be present and aware every moment as your life plays out.

PROGRESSIVE MUSCLE RELAXATION

The goal of progressive muscle relaxation is to notice the difference between tension and relaxed states in the body. This relaxation technique relieves pain by releasing tension in the neck and shoulders as well as the lower back. Just as cognitive therapy gives you the tools for psychological observation, this technique provides you with a means to observe your physical state. By practicing this technique, you will learn to recognize states of tension in your body. Progressive muscle relaxation does not require a big-time investment. Three daily sessions of just five minutes can have a significant effect in just three weeks.

Practice this meditation in a warm room because muscles do not relax as efficiently in a cool environment. It is best to do this technique before eating, so that your blood flow is not directed to your digestion.

When you are first learning this technique, lie on the floor so that your muscles are completely supported. Let your arms and legs rotate out. Place your hands on your stomach or at your sides. Make sure you are comfortable. You might want to use a small pillow under your neck or knees. As you progress, you will be able to do this relaxation technique while sitting or standing.

Progressive muscle relaxation deals with sixteen muscle groups. You will focus first on your hands and arms, starting with your dominant hand. You will move to your face, neck, body, and down to your feet. This first step is to contract a muscle group, producing a good deal of tension, then to release that tension all at once, which will create a momentum that will cause the muscles to relax more deeply. Relax as much as you tense, like a pendulum swinging side to side. Your relaxation will be deeper because of this momentum. If you feel pain in an area you are tensing, skip it and move on.

This is a very straightforward technique. There are only a few steps:

- Take a deep breath and hold it before you tense a muscle group.
- When you contract a muscle group, focus all your attention on those muscles.
- Tense the muscle group with as much force as you can. Hold the contraction for about five seconds.
- Notice the tightness and what tension feels like in those muscles.
- Let all the tension go.
- Notice how good those muscles feel. Breathe slowly for thirty seconds.
- Repeat the process with the same muscle group on the other side. Then move on to the next part of your body.

The chart that follows describes the way to tense and relax various areas of your body.

Muscles	How to Tense
Right hand and forearm	Make a tight fist with your upper arm relaxed.
Right upper arm	Press your elbows down against the floor or chair.
Left hand and forearm	Repeat the same movement as right hand and forearm.
Left upper arm	Repeat the same movement as right upper arm.
Forehead	Raise your eyebrows as high as possible.
Upper cheeks and nose	Wrinkle your nose and squint your eyes.
Lower face	Clench your jaw and smirk.
Neck	Try to raise and lower your chin at the same time.
Shoulders and neck	Raise your shoulders as if trying to touch your ears.
Chest, shoulders, upper back	Take a deep breath and pull your shoulder blades together.
Abdomen	Try to push your stomach out and pull it in at the same time.
Right thigh	Contract the large muscles on the front of your leg and the smaller muscles underneath. Press your heel down on the floor.
Right calf	Point the toes of your right foot, then flex your foot back with your toes pointing toward your knee.

Right foot	Point your toes, turn your foot in, and curl your toes gently.
Left thigh	Repeat same movements as right thigh.
Left calf	Repeat same movements as right calf.
Left foot	Repeat same movements as right foot.

If you have some hot spots, you can target them during the day, for example:

- If your neck and shoulders are tense or ache, you can reduce that tension by lifting your shoulders up to your ears and relaxing them several times.

- If you are holding tension in your core by holding your stomach muscles rigidly, pull those muscles in even more tightly, pressing your lower back to the chair or the floor. If you are standing, tilt your pelvis forward and release your stomach muscles.

- If you are breathing shallowly, press your shoulders back to expand your chest and inhale deeply.

- If you are grinding your teeth or furrowing your brow, you can work on the face moves.

Where the body holds tension is different for everyone. Doing the full progression will allow you to measure the level of relaxation you achieve in trouble spots as compared to other areas. This is how to train yourself to melt tension from your body. When you can release tension, your muscles will stop sending stress signals to your brain, which will extinguish or diminish your body's stress response and your experience of pain.

BODY SCAN MEDITATION

After you learn progressive muscle relaxation, you will be able to do a spot check on the tension levels in your body. Body scanning is a quick version of progressive muscle relaxation. Becoming aware of where your body is tense several times a day can help you to break the cycle of physical and psychological tension that can feed on itself. Breaking that cycle can reduce inflammation and improve sleep.

You can practice a simple scan anytime you feel stress or at random times throughout the day. This is how you do it:

- Sit comfortably or lie down. Some people like to do a body scan before falling asleep.

- Take a few deep belly breaths.

- Bring your attention to your feet. Observe sensations in your feet. If you notice pain, acknowledge it along with accompanying thoughts and emotions. Breathe through it.

- If you notice uncomfortable sensations, focus your attention on them. Breathe into them and observe what happens. Visualize the tension leaving your body through your breath and evaporating into the air. Move on when you feel ready.

- Continue doing this with each area of your body, moving up from your feet to the top of your head. Notice where you are feeling stress, tightness, pain, or pressure and breathe into it. This will help you to release the tension and enable you to recognize where stress is residing in your body in the future.

You can do an abbreviated version of this meditation by sitting and noticing a specific place in your body that is holding tension rather than moving from part to part. Learning to release muscle tension in this way will help you to manage your pain.

I have intentionally selected direct and simple meditations for you to introduce you to meditation. If you are having difficulty settling in or want to advance your practice, you might want to try a guided meditation. You can download many different meditations and apps that will inspire you and deepen your experience. I have produced *Lift: Meditations to Boost Back Health*, six audio meditations available wherever music and books are sold. If you would like to try a sample, go to DrKen.Hearnow.com where you will find excerpts of guided meditations that you can download.

You have now been introduced to the nine strategies of the Watch Your Back program. I know there is a lot to take in. You might be overwhelmed with the thought of trying to fit all the recommendations into your life. Do not let any negative chatter in your head divert you from trying to do all you can to reduce your pain and regain your vitality. The following chapter puts it all together in two daily programs that suggest a way to do it all and still have a life.

Chapter 13

The Watch Your Back Program: Putting It All Together

Y ou can take good care of your spine every day. In this chapter, I put it all together. It might seem overwhelming to incorporate all the strategies for taking good care of your spine each day. Showing you how a typical day looks on the Watch Your Back program demonstrates that the nine strategies can fit into your life without much trouble. The issue is to make these practices habitual, almost ritualistic. Of course, life happens, and a day can get disrupted. But it is only a morning, an afternoon, an evening, or a day. You can pick up where you left off and get right back on track.

I have created two programs: one for an early bird/morning person and another for a night owl/night person. The Watch Your Back program takes your natural biorhythms into account, which will make it easy to follow the program. I have estimated times of day to show how a day can flow. You will have to personalize the programs for your own schedule.

Early birds tend to be high-energy when they wake up, ready to hit the road running. Because they get up early, they have more time to themselves before the day officially begins. Morning people often slump mid-afternoon and before dinner. After a long day, they find it hard to keep their eyes open after a certain hour and usually turn in early.

Night owls burn the midnight oil and have a tough time getting out of bed in the morning. Time to themselves before work or when the demands of the day kick in is limited. Getting out of the house in the morning is often a fire drill. Their energy tends to peak when morning people fade.

Getting seven to eight hours of sleep is a challenge for them, especially if they have to start their day at a set time. They have to force themselves to go to bed to squeeze in enough restorative sleep.

If the daily schedule seems too daunting, you may want to ease into the program. One strategy may have special appeal for you because it answers a conscious need. Maybe you are sedentary and need to start moving. You could have a terrible time getting enough sleep and be desperate to try anything that will help you sleep well. Or you recognize that you are addicted to junk food and need to clean up your act when it comes to what you eat. Your negative view of things might get you down, and you could be stressed out all the time. Positive thinking and meditation could lift you up and calm you down. If your chronic back pain is exhausting you, doing the stretches and progressive muscle relaxation could make a big difference.

The idea is to commit to trying something. If you incorporate one or two strategies into your life, you will notice a difference and want to try more. If the strategy does not deliver what you expect, see if another works better for you. As soon as one strategy becomes a habit, move on to another.

Or you could jump right in and follow the program, which is not as demanding as you might think. You do not have to spend hours at the gym or sitting on a mat meditating for long stretches of time. In a little over fifty minutes, broken up into small segments throughout the day, you can do the entire program.

Taking care to watch your back will raise your energy, turn down your pain, and increase your well-being immeasurably.

EARLY BIRD/MORNING PERSON

Wake-Up Routine

6:00

Wake up at the same time every day.

Practice positivity: Rather than being anxious about the day ahead, think about all you will accomplish and what you want to achieve. (2 minutes)

Stretches: Begin the day by doing a few stretches. Select three or four stretches depending on where you are feeling stiff or sore. (Pages 86–93) (3 minutes)

Watch Your Back Workout: Begin with the six exercises in Workout 1. This will energize you for the day ahead. (Pages 167–172) (10 to 20 minutes)

Before the Day Begins

6:30 Supplements and Water

Stay hydrated: Your goal is to drink roughly eight eight-ounce glasses of water a day. To ensure that you do so, make it a habit to drink a glass of water every odd hour.

Healthy breakfast: Your early start may give you the time to prepare a good, nutritious meal to launch your day and build in a bit of time for yourself.

7:00 Aerobic Activity

Go for a walk, a bike ride, a swim, or do yoga or Pilates from an online class before work or after the children leave for school. (10 to 30 minutes depending on how much time you have)

Shower and dress.

9:00–5:00

Get up and move twice every hour: Whether you work at a desk, run a household, or drive around town delivering packages, remind yourself that being sedentary for hours is bad for your back and your overall health.

10:30 Mid-Morning Anywhere, Anytime Stretches

Read your body and select three or four exercises to loosen up. (Pages 135–153) (2 minutes)

Healthy snack: This pick-me-up will delay hunger pangs and keep your energy on an even keel. (Pages 197–198)

Noon

Posture Correcting Stretches: Evaluate how you have been sitting or standing to identify posture mistakes and areas of your body that are tense. Select three or four posture stretches to relax your muscles. (Pages 86–93) (3 minutes)

Healthy lunch.

Aerobics: Try to fit in a walk before or after you eat. (Pages 127–131) (10 minutes)

Get up and move: Avoid being sedentary for long periods by standing and moving twice every hour.

3:00 Mid-afternoon

Deep breathing: If your energy is starting to lag or you are losing concentration, belly breathing will renew your energy and focus. (2 minutes)

Healthy snack: Dinner will not be for hours. Nourishing your body now will help you to resist snacking before dinner.

5:00–5:30 End of the Workday

Posture Correcting Stretches: Choose three or four exercises to relieve your body of pent-up tension. (Pages 86–93 (2 minutes)

5:30–6:00 After Work/Before Dinner

Meditate: You have been awake almost twelve hours at this point. This is a good time to re-center before your evening begins. (Start with 2 minutes and increase to 20)

Dinner

Try to eat at least three hours before you want to go to sleep.

9:30–10:00 Bedtime Routine

Do something to wind down: It could be catching up on magazines, reading a book, listening to music, taking a bath, anything that is a treat for you.

Go to bed the same time every night: You want to make sure you get seven or eight hours of good sleep.

Practice positivity: Think of the good things that happened and what you accomplished that day. If your day was less than perfect, look at what went wrong in a good light. Be confident that you will do better next time. Review all the things you are grateful for. (3 minutes)

Deep calming breathing: This will relax you and allow your mind and body to let go of the stress of the day. (2 minutes)

NIGHT OWL/NIGHT PERSON

Wake-Up Routine

8:00

Wake up at the same time every day. Because you tend to stay in bed as long as you can, your activities are minimal before the day begins.

Posture Correcting Stretches: Get the kinks out and your energy flowing as soon as you are out of bed. Select three or four stretches depending on where you are feeling stiff or sore. (Pages 86–93) (3 minutes)

Deep breathing: Fire up your body with a boost from belly breathing. (2 minutes)

Before the Day Begins

Shower and dress: Put yourself together for the day. Take the stress out what you are going to wear by making your selections the night before.

Supplements and water: Stay hydrated. Your goal is to drink roughly eight eight-ounce glasses of water a day. To ensure that you do, make it a habit to drink a glass of water every odd hour.

Quick healthy breakfast: Planning ahead makes sense if you are short on time. Whether you have breakfast at home or pick up something on the way to work, advance planning will help you to avoid grabbing a sweet, high carb breakfast.

9:00–5:00

Get up and move twice every hour: Whether you work at a desk, run a household, or you drive around to deliver packages, remind yourself to get up and move every hour. Sitting or being sedentary for hours is bad for your back and overall health.

10:30 Mid-Morning Anywhere, Anytime Stretches

Read your body to find the tense spots. Select three or four exercises to loosen up. (Pages 135–153) (2 minutes)

Healthy snack. (Pages 197–198)

Noon

Posture Correcting Stretches: Evaluate your posture as you have been sitting or standing. Choose three or four exercises to relieve your body of pent-up tension. (Pages 86–93) (3 minutes)

Aerobics: Carve out time mid-day to take a walk, bike, swim, go to a gym, take a Pilates or yoga class. Exercising before lunch will help you avoid over-indulging. If you are too busy during the day, do something that gets you moving after work or before dinner. (15–30 minutes)

Healthy lunch.

3:00 Mid-Afternoon

Deep breathing: Time to take a pause to refresh yourself. (3 minutes)

Posture Correcting Stretches: Choose three to loosen up. (Pages 86–93) (3 minutes)

Healthy snack: Dinner will not be for hours. Nourishing your body now will help you to avoid snacking before dinner. (Pages 197–198)

5:30–6:00 After Work/Before Dinner

Watch Your Back Workout: Begin with the six exercises in Workout 1. This will be a great break between the demands of the day and the start of the evening. (Pages 167–172) (10 to 20 minutes)

Practice positivity: Think about all you have accomplished during the day. If you have had some bumpy spots, think about how you could have reacted or handled them differently. (3 minutes)

Dinner

Try to eat at least three hours before you want to go to sleep.

12:30 Bedtime Routine

Do something to wind down: Ease into your bedtime routine by doing something you enjoy, such as reading a book or magazine, listening to music or a podcast—anything that is a treat for you.

Practice positivity: Review all that went well during the day and be thankful for the good things in your life. Consider how you have reacted differently to annoyances and disappointments. Think about what you hope tomorrow will be like. (3 minutes)

Meditation: Meditating before going to bed will help you to wind down and defuse negativity. (Begin with 2 minutes and increase to 20)

Deep breathing before bed: This will further relax you and allow your mind and body to release the stress of the day. (2 minutes)

Go to bed at the same time every night: Decide on a time that will allow you seven or eight hours of restorative sleep and stick with it.

Chapter 14

Extra Help

I often advise patients to support the Watch Your Back program with complementary medicine and alternative approaches, which can sometimes help to speed healing and relieve pain. In some cases, I stage a full-on campaign with a team of healthcare professionals to supplement and support my treatment. Do you know what a physiatrist (a DO or an MD), an osteopathic physician (a DO), a chiropractor (a DC), or a physical therapist (a PT or DPT) does and how they differ? You are not alone. Most people are confused about their training and roles. Before I describe various alternative therapies, I want to explain the focus of each of these healthcare professions and what each does to treat pain and spine problems.

HEALTHCARE PROFESSIONALS TO HELP WATCH YOUR BACK

A physiatrist is a Physical Medicine and Rehabilitation (PM&R) physician, who has completed a bachelor's degree followed by four years of medical school and four years of a post-doctoral residency. They are medical doctors who have completed training in sub-specialties that include sports medicine, neuromuscular, spinal cord injury, and pain medicine, to name a few. They treat conditions affecting the brain, spinal cord, nerves, bones, joints, ligaments, muscles, and tendons. Physiatrists' treatment is focused on function and the musculoskeletal system. They diagnose and treat the cause of pain and/or dysfunction, with the goals of decreasing pain, recovering mobility, preventing further disability, and maximizing function. Back pain is their focus because the spine is the center of the musculoskeletal system. Their treatments include assessment of medications, spine, muscle, and joint injections, nerve stimulation, bracing, and post-operative rehabilitation.

Osteopaths, chiropractors, and physical therapists all focus on non-invasive, drug-free, manual techniques. They all perform soft tissue manipulation, massage, stretching muscle groups, and spine adjustments.

Osteopathic physicians first complete their bachelor's degree, followed by four years of medical school to earn their doctor of osteopathy degree (DO), which is then followed with a post-doctoral residency of their choice, from family practice and pediatrics to radiology and orthopedic surgery. The medical academic curriculum is virtually the same as an allopathic physician (MD). Osteopathic physicians do an extra 200 hours of course work in hands-on diagnosing and treatment. This allows DOs to have extra armamentarium in their doctor's bag to treat the patient as a whole. The primary osteopathic principles are the interconnectedness of mind, body, and spirit, the body's ability to heal itself, and the interrelationship between the body's function and structure.

Osteopathic Manipulative Treatments (OMT) such as stretching, gentle pressure, and resistance aim to improve overall health by manipulating and strengthening the musculoskeletal framework; they focus on the structure of the body and how it functions. An osteopathic physician focuses on the fascia, joints, muscles, and spine. Wellness oriented, their philosophy is that posture, injury, and lifestyle patterns can compromise the body's anatomical structure, resulting in poor health. An osteopathic physician may use OMT alone or in combination with medications, surgery, rehabilitation, diet, and exercise.

Chiropractors and physical therapists may focus on non-invasive, drug-free manual techniques. They perform soft tissue manipulation, massage, stretching muscle groups, and spine adjustments.

Chiropractors earn a Doctor of Chiropractic degree (DC) in a four-year program after completing four years of an undergraduate degree. The requirements do vary state-to-state. The philosophy of chiropractic theory is that the proper alignment of the body's musculoskeletal structure, the spine in particular, enables the body to heal itself without surgery or medication. Chiropractors use hands-on spinal manipulation and other alternative treatments.

Manipulation is used to restore mobility to joints restricted by injury caused by a traumatic event or repetitive stress—sitting without proper back support, for example. Chiropractic treatment is primarily used as a pain relief alternative for muscles, joints, bones, and connective tissue, such as cartilage, ligaments, and tendons. Spinal manipulation to treat low back pain is documented to be safe and effective, especially in the hands of a properly trained practitioner. A chiropractor may employ modalities such as hot or cold packs, stimulation, massage, and exercise regimens to help to rehabilitate the spine. Chiropractors are involved in the use of proper posture to help people.

Physical therapists earn a Doctor of Physical Therapy (DPT) degree in a three-year program after a bachelor's degree. Physical therapy can be called physiotherapy. Some practitioners suggest that physiotherapy is more concerned with manual therapy. The therapist helps to improve the patient's injury with a hands-on approach by stretching, soft tissue release, joint mobilizations, and fascial release. Physical therapy is a more exercise-based approach that teaches patients exercises to strengthen muscles, improve balance, and sharpen coordination. In fact, in the United States, the terms can be used interchangeably, and most physical therapy practices combine the two approaches. The focus of physical therapy is on the prevention of injury, the improvement of flexibility, and the management of acute pain.

COMPLEMENTARY THERAPIES FOR BACK PAIN

My holistic approach to helping my patients manage their pain includes introducing them to alternatives to traditional, mainstream medical treatments. To give you an idea of the available options, this chapter describes alternative therapies that can support your efforts to take control of your pain and improve the health of your spine. As always, check with your doctor before trying one of these therapies. When you are selecting someone to administer the treatments make sure the person is professionally certified.

Spinal Manipulation and Mobilization

Osteopathic physicians, who perform OMT in their practice, and chiropractors manually adjust the spine to improve joint mobility and reduce pain. Spinal manipulation may involve a technique known as a high-velocity, low-amplitude thrust that produces the cracking sound associated with a chiropractic adjustment. Otherwise, spinal mobilization involves slow, firm movements of the spinal joints through their full range of motion. The treatment is used for sciatica, lower back and neck pain, and headaches. Before undergoing spinal manipulation, be sure you do not have a serious underlying condition, for example, a spinal fracture, herniated disc, osteoporosis, spinal cord compression, inflammatory arthritis, or if you are pregnant or taking blood-thinning medication.

Cranial Therapy (CT)

This therapy, which is also known as craniosacral therapy (CST), is a type of bodywork that relieves compression in the bones of the head, sacrum (a triangular bone in the lower back), and the spinal column. CT uses gentle pressure on the head, neck, and back to relieve the stress and pain caused by compression. This can soothe pain and release emotional and physical stress and tension. The theory is that the gentle manipulation of the bones in the skull, spine, and pelvis normalizes the flow of cerebrospinal fluid in the central nervous system. Removing blockages from the normal flow is said to increase the body's ability to heal. Massage therapists, physical therapists, some osteopathic physicians, and chiropractors can perform this treatment. Craniosacral therapy is used as a treatment for headaches and migraines, insomnia and disturbed sleep cycles, and neck pain, to name a few conditions. The treatment should not be used for those with severe bleeding disorders, an aneurysm, or a history of recent head injuries. I often recommend CT for people who are extremely stressed. My patients have found this therapy very effective. These treatments produce an intense feeling of deep relaxation, reset muscle fibers, break pain and stress cycles, and allow the body to restore and heal itself.

Massage

Massage has many benefits for people with acute and chronic back pain. In addition to the psychological benefit of relaxation, the treatment stimulates the production of endorphins. The mood enhancers can ease depression and anxiety, which helps to reduce pain. Endorphins increase blood flow and circulation, which brings nutrition to muscles and tissues. This aids recovery from muscle soreness and strain. Massage decreases tension in the muscles, which can improve sleep and flexibility and reduces pain caused by tight muscles. Massage is an effective treatment for muscle strain in the lower and upper back, neck, and spinal arthritis.

Research indicates that moderate-intensity massage offers more pain relief than light-touch massage. Massage not only gets out the knots from your muscles but also manipulates lactic acid and lymphatic drainage in your body. A sore back can result from the buildup of lactic acid or waste products in your muscles. Massage moves lactic acid quickly from your muscles, which helps your body to heal faster.

Forty-four states in addition to the District of Columbia, Puerto Rico, and the U.S. Virgin Islands have a certification process that requires a license, which must be renewed on a regular basis. The majority of licenses require continuing education for renewal. When selecting a massage therapist, check the requirements in your state and the credentials of the therapist.

There are so many different types of massage that it is hard to pick the right one for you. I will make that choice easier by describing nine massages that are good for pain relief.

- **Swedish Massage** is a gentle full-body massage, which helps to release knots in your muscles, promotes relaxation, and boosts circulation. The therapist uses a combination of long, flowing strokes in the direction of the heart, kneading, and passive joint movement. You may experience mild to moderate pain.

- **Deep Tissue Massage** uses more pressure than a Swedish massage, relieving tension in the deeper layers of muscle tissue. This type of massage is ideal for releasing chronic tension and is said to improve range of motion. If you suffer from chronic aches and pains, tight muscles, and anxiety, this massage is for you.

- **Shiatsu Massage** is a Japanese style of massage based on Chinese medicine. The goal is to eliminate blockages that keep the body's energy force, called Qi (pronounced "Chee"), from flowing freely. Shiatsu massage therapists use a variety of techniques, using their elbows, knees, and feet as they work out tension from the back, joints, and limbs. The therapist might focus on areas of your body that need attention. This technique promotes relaxation and calm, relieves stress, anxiety, and depression, and reduces muscle tension. You can be fully clothed during this massage.

- **Sports Massage** is a variation on Swedish massage that aims to address aches caused by repetitive motion and help active people make a quick recovery from stress and injury. This technique promotes speedier recovery times, a better range of motion, and improved performance. It can be used to relieve pain, anxiety, and muscle tension. This can be a full-body massage, or the therapist may focus on the part of the body needing attention. You can keep your clothes on for this massage.

- **Trigger Point Massage** dispels chronic tension located deep in the muscle. Trigger points are areas of tightness in muscle tissue that can cause pain in other parts of the body. By focusing on relieving trigger points, this type of massage can reduce pain and is especially effective for sciatica and stiff joints. Warning: trigger point massage has a reputation of being a bit painful.

- **Hot Stone Massage** is similar to Swedish massage except the massage therapist uses heated basalt stones on different areas of your body, particularly the back, to help melt tight areas. Therapists can hold a stone as they massage your body using gentle Swedish massage techniques. The heat from the stones can also improve blood flow and relieve muscle tension.

- **Aromatherapy Massage** has an emotional healing component. The technique combines gentle pressure with the use of essential oils, which are diluted before being applied to the skin. While you are being massaged, you will inhale essential oils diffused in the air and absorb them through your skin. Aromatherapy massage can help to boost your mood, relieve symptoms of depression, and relieve pain and muscle tension.

- **Thai Massage** is an active form of massage. It works the entire body using a sequence of movements like yoga stretches. The therapist will use palms and fingers to apply firm pressure to your body. You will be stretched and twisted in various positions. This massage reduces and relieves pain and stress, increases flexibility, improves circulation, and raises energy levels. You are fully clothed, but it is best to wear comfortable, loose clothing for this type of massage.

- **Prenatal Massage** aims to relieve pregnancy pains, stress, muscle tension, and insomnia for expecting mothers. Instead of lying on her back, the pregnant woman either reclines on her side or uses a massage table with a hole cut in it that allows her to recline on her stomach. You can get this type of massage at any time during your pregnancy, but many facilities advise women in their first trimester not to get one. The therapist focuses on the lower back, hips, and legs.

If the descriptions of these massage treatments do not make you want to find a good massage therapist immediately, you should read them again. If you have not had a massage before, it is hard to describe the sensations you will experience during the massage and the level of relaxation you will feel after. You will leave the massage table feeling in touch with your body. Having a massage is a rewarding way to practice mindfulness.

Acupuncture

Acupuncture is one of the best alternative treatments for back pain. The treatment is especially helpful if you have muscle spasms or nerve-related pain. This ancient Chinese treatment is designed to unblock and move the body's energy, called Qi ("Chee"), through the body's systems. This energy flow, or vital force, can be stimulated to create balance and health. The energy flows through the body along twelve main channels known as meridians. The meridians represent the major organs and functions of the body, though they do not follow the exact pathways of nerves or blood flow.

The goal of acupuncture is to correct imbalances of flow and restore health through stimulations. This is achieved by inserting thin needles through the skin at points along the meridians of the body. If you are worried about the needles, I have to assure you that the procedure is pain-less. By stimulating the proper points, parts of the nervous system are stimulated to relieve pain. Some acupuncture points for lower back pain include points on the back of the knees, feet, lower back, hands, hips, and stomach. For upper back pain, the points are located in the head, neck, shoulders, and upper back.

The way acupuncture works is not completely understood, but it is thought to work for back pain by:

- Stimulating the nervous system to release chemicals from the spinal cord, muscles, and brain, which are believed to be pain relieving.

- Releasing opioid-like chemicals produced in the body.

- Releasing neurotransmitters that send messages regulating the on/off mechanisms of nerve endings. Acupuncture is believed to stimulate some neurotransmitters that shut off pain.

- Triggering electromagnetic impulses in the body, which speeds up the way the body handles pain.

Forty-seven states and the District of Columbia have a certification pro-cess for acupuncturists. The requirements are not the same in all states. In some, a series of exams is part of the licensing process, in others a national certification is required along with the state license. For example, in New York State you must successfully complete exams through the National Certification Commission for Acupuncture and Oriental Medicine (NCCAOM), which include Acupuncture with Point Location and Foundations of Oriental Medicine. Before seeing an acupuncturist, check what is required in your state.

Biofeedback

Biofeedback is a treatment used to learn to control some of the body's functions. During biofeedback, you are connected to electrical sensors that show you information about your body on a screen. The sensors can be used to monitor your brainwaves, skin temperature, muscle tension, heart rate, and breathing. Biofeedback is a tool for increasing awareness and changing your physiological responses to reduce symptoms. The feedback, the data which appears on the screen, shows you what happens when you change your thoughts, emotions, or behavior. The treatment helps you to make subtle changes in your body, such as relaxing certain muscles. For example, biofeedback can pinpoint tense muscles that cause pain. With biofeedback you learn how to relax those specific muscles to reduce your pain.

You know that stress and pain can make each other worse. Posture and breathing habits can perpetuate pain. When you become aware of the habitual patterns, such as muscle tension or shallow breathing, that are contributing to your pain, you can try to change those habits, which will interrupt the pain-stress feedback loop.

One treatment goal for chronic pain sufferers is to reduce activation of the sympathetic nervous system, which regulates the stress response, and turn on the relaxation response of the parasympathetic nervous system. Biofeedback can teach you how to have more conscious control over each response. Being able to control your stress response is a powerful tool for managing chronic pain. Biofeedback can help with insomnia and anxiety as well.

Biofeedback is used by psychologists, physical therapists, occupational therapists, nurses, physicians, and other licensed healthcare professionals. You can receive biofeedback training in physical therapy clinics, medical centers, and hospitals. From interactive computer programs to wearable devices, many biofeedback devices are available for home use. The FDA has not approved or regulated many at-home devices. Before trying biofeedback therapy at home, discuss available devices with your healthcare team.

Transcutaneous Electrical Nerve Stimulation (TENS)

TENS uses a low voltage electrical current to provide pain relief. The unit consists of a battery-powered device that delivers electrical impulses through electrodes placed on the surface of your skin. The electrodes are placed at or near nerves where the pain is located or at trigger points. You feel a tingling sensation. The machine has a dial that allows you to control the strength of the electrical impulses.

Two theories explain how TENS works. One explanation is that the electric current stimulates nerve cells that block the transmission of pain signals, which changes your perception of pain. The other theory is that nerve stimulation raises the level of endorphins, the body's natural painkillers, to block the perception of pain.

You can find TENS equipment, which is a small and portable unit, at a pain specialist, physiatrist, acupuncturist, orthopedist, or a physiotherapist center. You can buy your own TENS machine, but to get the most benefit from TENS it is important that the settings are adjusted correctly for you and your condition. You will need guidance about where to put the electrodes as well.

Do not use TENS or be very careful about electrode placement if you have an implantable device, are pregnant, have cancer, epilepsy, or deep vein thrombosis.

Yoga and Pilates

These schools of movement work on body symmetry for proper alignment, breathing, muscle strengthening, and flexibility, all of which are goals of the Watch Your Back program. In fact, many of the exercises in the program are yoga and Pilates moves. Pilates is designed to strengthen the core muscles and hips. Yoga targets the strength and flexibility of the spine as it creates a sense of calm and focus.

You might want to add a full Pilates or yoga class to your physical activities. I do advise caution if you have degenerated or herniated discs or a stress fracture because stretching the spine could be counterproductive. If you take a class, inform your instructor of any injuries you have. The rule of thumb is to start slowly and progress gradually.

You can find yoga and Pilates studios just about everywhere. You can choose from countless free apps, YouTube shows, and online downloads that offer yoga and Pilates sessions at every level. Try a few different ones to find the right one for you.

Herbal Remedies

Herbal remedies are an increasingly popular way to manage pain. Though research on herbal remedies is still in its early phases, many herbs, which have been used for millennia, are thought to provide pain management and decrease inflammation. Before trying any of these herbs to treat your pain, talk to your doctor. There may be side effects, or a particular herb could interact with a prescribed medicine. The best course is to talk to a healthcare professional before trying an herbal remedy.

The following eight herbs are believed to provide natural pain relief and to reduce inflammation:

- **Devil's claw:** Comes from southern Africa, where it has been used for centuries to treat fever, arthritis, and gastrointestinal problems. It works as an anti-inflammatory. It is available in capsule form.

- **White willow bark:** If you do not want to take the synthetic version, also known as aspirin, white willow bark helps with conditions that cause pain or inflammation. It is known to relieve acute back pain. You can find it in the form of tablets, capsules, powder, or liquid.

- **Capsaicin cream:** Capsaicin is what makes chili peppers hot. In topical form, it may help to relieve your pain. It is said to deplete a substance that conveys the pain sensation from the peripheral to the central nervous system. It can take several days for this to occur, so do not give up if it does not work right away. It reduces pain temporarily and needs to be re-applied four or five times a day. Wash hands well after applying.

- **Ginger:** Ginger extract is said to help with muscle and joint pain because it contains anti-inflammatory phytochemicals. You can find ginger as a powder, capsule, or tablet.

- **Feverfew:** Also called featherfew or bachelor's buttons. It is a medicinal plant that has been used for centuries to treat fever, migraines, arthritis, and tooth and stomach aches. Research has found that the flowers and leaves have pain-relieving properties. Feverfew contains compounds that may reduce inflammation and spasms. You can purchase feverfew in capsule, tablet, or liquid extract form.

- **Turmeric:** Contains an active ingredient called curcumin. It is said to reduce inflammation and have pain-relieving qualities. Supplements are available in a variety of forms.

- **St. John's wort:** A flowering shrub that has been used in the treatment of nervous disorders since ancient Greece. The active ingredient, hyperforin, has anti-bacterial, anti-viral, antioxidant, and anti-inflammatory properties. It is popularly used to treat mild to moderate depression. As a topical, St. John's wort helps to heal burns. It is said to relieve neuropathic pain as well as pain associated with arthritis and sciatica. It is sold as a tea, in tablet, liquid, and topical form. St. John's wort can cause serious interactions with some medications. Make sure to check if your medications are on the proscribed list.

- **Valerian root:** Used for centuries as a sleeping aid. Its calming qualities are said to reduce anxiety. As a pain reliever, it is especially effective for spasms and muscle cramps. It is available in powder, liquid, tea, or pills. If you have insomnia, this is the herb for you.

Going for extra help can support you and enable you to get even more from the Watch Your Back program. I have seen the lives of so many patients expand as their pain diminishes. Being in their bodies becomes a different experience. They are no longer held back by their pain. They become more adventurous, and with their renewed energy, try many things they never thought possible. Witnessing their exuberance is the greatest reward I could have as a physician. I want the same for you.

Afterword

Let Me Know How You Are Doing

W hen I first thought of designing a program to help my patients triumph over their pain, I sat at my computer late one night and randomly made a list of the advice I had doled out over the years. I was surprised by how far-reaching my recommendations were, though I should not have been. I have spent endless hours reading the results of new studies on back pain. Being familiar with the latest findings could be a full-time job, but I know that being on top of what is happening in my field is one of the best ways I can make a difference in my patients' lives. As I watched so many of my patients begin to take a more active role in managing their pain, I knew I had to develop a plan of action that could work for anyone.

I sorted through my list, then thought about the success stories in my practice. I was able to isolate the characteristics, attitudes, and behavior changes behind the dramatic improvements I had witnessed. That is how the nine strategies came to be. The Watch Your Back program soon followed. I could see transformations in patients whose lives had been defined and constrained by chronic pain. Their lives, once narrow, opened up to boundless possibilities. Hearing from them about their progress means a great deal to me.

I know that *Watch Your Back* covers a lot of ground. I wanted to expose you to a full-blown examination of what works to prevent or reduce back pain. I have included scientific explanations because I believe that knowing the program is based in real science helps you in making a commitment. This book is not offering you a magic-bullet solution. You will not see a miracle in seven days. The program is not something you do until the pain goes away. You do not go "on" and "off" the program. In order to defeat chronic pain, you have to be willing to change your life in significant ways. Though the strategies may seem challenging, trying to convert harmful habits to healing ones has got to be more rewarding than living in pain.

To help you, I have created an interactive website at DrKen.us to provide a blog and my podcast *All Things Spine*, in which I interview industry leaders to emphasize the key points of the Watch Your Back program. Please enjoy the free content and sign in to let us know how you are doing and progressing.

Based on my years of meditation and thinking about helping people with back pain, I created a series of meditations called *Lift: Meditations to Boost Back Health*. The "My Genius Brain" meditation encourages you to respect the words of your genius brain. The "Deep Belly Breathing and Tensionometer Meditation" explains the importance of deep belly breathing and how the technique is practiced. This meditation introduces the concept of the neck, back, and head tensionometer. "Posture Forces on the Spine" is a neuro-linguistic programming meditation (left ear, right ear, and center channel) meant to help bring awareness to your posture, especially to the everyday postural forces, such as text neck, belly fat, breast weight, lifting, and backpack forces. The "10 Free Physicians" meditation recognizes that people around the world are looking for ways to stop pain without narcotics. This meditation conspires to make you happy, healthy, and pain free by focusing on techniques you have in your own hands to feel better and do more. The meditation introduces you to ten free physicians who will help you to get rid of pain: mental well-being, meditation, thinking, nutrition, posture, breath, range of motion, strength, sleep, and attire. The "Lift: Who Am I" meditation reveals that an average person lifts twenty to fifty pounds per day, which is 5,000 to 18,000 pounds a year. Some delivery people lift 1 to 1.5 million pounds per year. The "Lift: My Daily Routine" meditation is directed to people who lift for a living. The meditation provides a daily protocol for readiness, including breath work, stretch work, strength work, aerobic work, and my half-hour vacation. *Lift: Meditations to Boost Back Health* is available wherever songs and books are sold.

When you commit to watching your back, you will be putting your life on a new trajectory toward health, renewed vitality, and a feeling of overall well-being. I hope the Watch Your Back program can transform your life, as it has for so many of my patients. Please let me know how you are doing. I would love to hear about your successes and challenges. You can contact me at KKH@DrKen.us.

Acknowledgments

To my great co-writer, Diane Reverand, for her brilliant mind, dedication to health, and excellence in writing.

To my agent, Marilyn Allen, for her untiring enthusiasm, skills, work, and creativity to help me to share my message and mission with millions of people worldwide.

To Haven Iverson and Jade Lascelles, my superb editors at Sounds True Books, and the entire Sounds True team, including Nick Small, our publicity expert, book placement and distribution experts, the sales representatives, and Chloé Prusiewicz with her marketing team for your immense efforts to help people with back pain. And to copyeditor Brent Smith, proofreaders Suzanne Najarian and Bridget Manzella, and indexer Jeff Hoffman for your thorough assistance.

To my amazing wife, Physical Medicine and Rehabilitation specialist Dr. Marcia Griffin-Hansraj, for your thousands of discussions and edits.

To my friend and genius illustrator, Gary Crumpler, who rendered these stylish, transparent black and white 2.5D illustrations.

To public relation specialists Shay Pantano & Richard Rubenstein, who are instrumental in spreading these messages worldwide.

To my friend Richard Rubenstein, who has guided me each step of the way.

To my parents, my brother and sisters Mark, Jan, Lynn, Ann, Camille, and my nephew Chad Agrawal for your encouragement that nothing is impossible.

To Brenda Griffin for your spiritual support and for reminding me to be my best self every day.

To all of my professors in life, including Briggs Persaud, Dr. Chitranjan Ranawat, Dr. Patrick O'Leary, Dr. Frank Cammisa, Dr. Oheneba Boachie-Adjei, Dr. Lance Weaver, Dr. John Chiu, Dr. David Payne, and Dr. Gregory Chiaramonte.

To Jacqueline Reeder for twenty years of service safely preparing patients for spine surgery, to the operating room staff, anesthesiologists, nurses, and healthcare workers who have helped me to render spine care.

To my mastermind partners, Iman Mutlaq and Ninad Tipnis, for your enduring friendship and planning projects of new heights.

To my dear patients who have inspired me to write the messages to help people everywhere.

List of Exercises

CHAPTER 4

Posture Correcting Stretches/Posture Fixes

CHAPTER 7

Anywhere, Anytime Stretches

The Life Aquatic

CHAPTER 8

The Workouts

Workout 1

Workout 2

Index

About the Author

D r. Ken Hansraj is a spinal and orthopedic surgeon with more than 20 years' experience who focuses on the whole body and preventative care. Board certified by the American Board of Orthopedic Surgery, he is double fellowship trained in spine surgery and biomechanics at the Hospital for Special Surgery in New York. Dr. Hansraj specializes in spine surgery, using minimally invasive approaches to spinal care whenever possible, and he has developed a breakthrough strategy using stem cells for failed spinal surgeries. He has appeared on CNN, CBS, Fox, NBC, ABC, and NPR. He was named one of America's most compassionate doctors in 2020 by Vitals.com and is frequently rated as one of New York's top doctors. He lives with his wife and son in Rockland County, New York.

About Sounds True

Sounds True is a multimedia publisher whose mission is to inspire and support personal transformation and spiritual awakening. Founded in 1985 and located in Boulder, Colorado, we work with many of the leading spiritual teachers, thinkers, healers, and visionary artists of our time. We strive with every title to preserve the essential "living wisdom" of the author or artist. It is our goal to create products that not only provide information to a reader or listener but also embody the quality of a wisdom transmission.

For those seeking genuine transformation, Sounds True is your trusted partner. At SoundsTrue.com you will find a wealth of free resources to support your journey, including exclusive weekly audio interviews, free downloads, interactive learning tools, and other special savings on all our titles.

To learn more, please visit SoundsTrue.com/freegifts or call us toll-free at 800.333.9185.

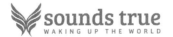